complete
massage
A Visual Guide to Over 100 Techniques

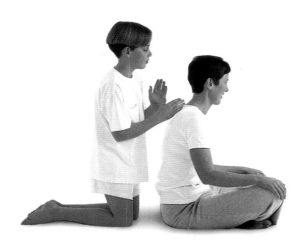

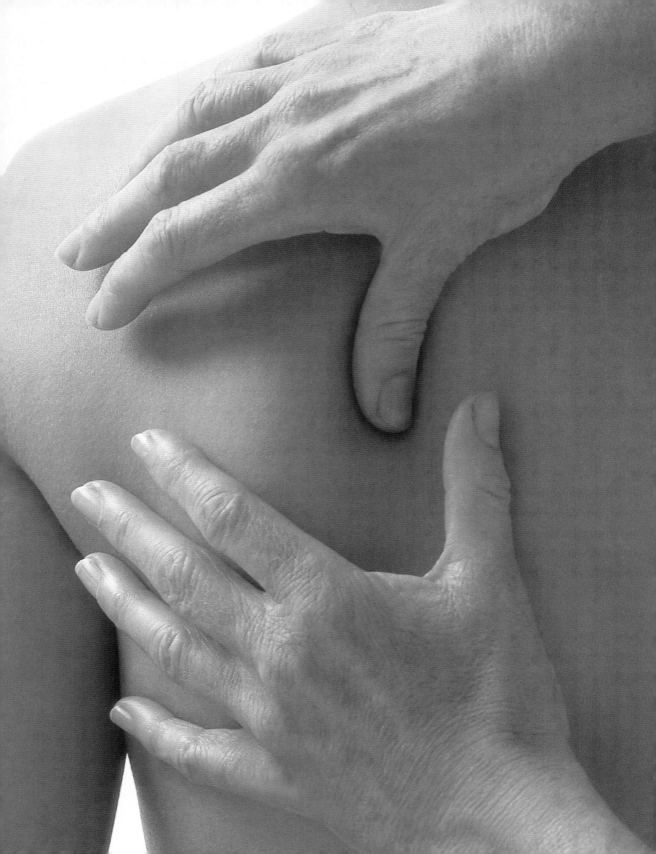

complete
massage

A Visual Guide to Over 100 Techniques

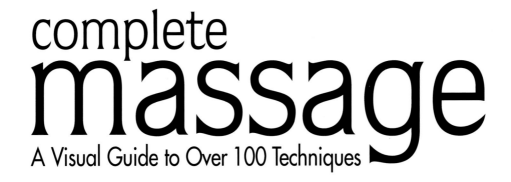

Clare Maxwell-Hudson

Massage photography
Sandra Lousada

A DK Publishing Book

LONDON, NEW YORK, MUNICH, MELBOURNE and DELHI

Project Editors: Monica Chakraverty, Nell Graville

Art Editors: Helen Diplock, Carole Perks

Designer: Rachana Shah

Senior Art Editor: Tracey Clarke

Managing Editors: Mary Ling, Susannah Marriott

Managing Art Editor: Toni Kay

Senior Managing Editor: Krystyna Mayer

DTP Designer: Karen Ruane

Digital Image Manipulation: Bridget Roseberry

Production Manager: Maryann Webster

*This book is gratefully dedicated
to Shah, Mina and Gill.*

First American Edition, 1999
4 6 8 10 9 7 5 3

First published in Great Britain in 1999
by Dorling Kindersley Limited,
375 Hudson Street
New York, New York, 10014

Published in the United States by
DK Publishing, Inc.,
375 Hudson Street
New York, New York, 10014

This paperback edition published 2001
Copyright © 1999, 2001 Dorling Kindersley Limited
Text copyright © 1999, 2001 Clare Maxwell-Hudson
Massage photography © 1999, 2001 Sandra Lousada

A Cataloging-in-Publication record is available from
the Library of Congress

ISBN 978-0-7984-7990-5

Reproduced by Colourscan, Singapore
Printed in Singapore by Star Standard
D.L.TO:819-2002

see our complete product line at
www.dk.com

Important Notice
Refer to the safety precautions on pages 14 and 16 before
commencing a massage. If you are in any doubt as to whether to
massage an area, seek a physician's advice first. Refer to the cautions
on pages 14–15 before using any essential oil. Neither the author nor
the publisher can be held responsible for any damage, injury, or
otherwise resulting from the use of massage or essential oils.

CONTENTS

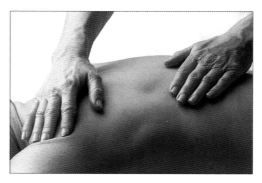

GALLERY OF STROKES

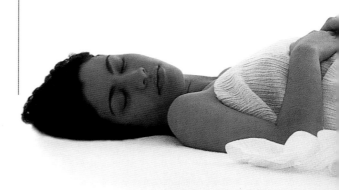

INTRODUCTION

MOST PEOPLE LOVE TO TRAVEL, and most people also love to be massaged, so you can imagine how incredibly lucky I feel that my life contains both these delights. Since I first trained in London and Paris, I have visited many parts of the world, searching out massage techniques and the many ways people help each other through touch.

My first journey was actually done in the library of the British Museum, where I sat researching day after day, tracking massage back over the centuries and finding it everywhere, from Polynesia to Persia, from Japan to the Sandwich Islands. I learned how in ancient Greece, Herodicus, teacher of Hippocrates, the father of Western medicine, made massage and exercise a cornerstone of the medicine of the day – something that modern doctors now support. In ancient Rome, Cicero, the great orator, said he owed as much to his "anointer" as to his physician, and Julius Caesar was "pinched" daily by a specially trained slave, to alleviate his neuralgic pains. In the 6th century, the physician Aetius of Amide ordered massage for certain women "who do not conceive." This is just what we are beginning to do again today; recently I have come across two cases of massage used on women with this problem, and both later successfully conceived.

After traveling through history, my real journeys began. In places as diverse as America and Afghanistan, New Zealand and Zanzibar, the *hammams* of Turkey and Hungary and mountain villages in Thailand, I learned everything I could. I found that while we in the West work with anatomy and physiology in mind, in the East, people work with the concept of balancing energy in the body. I was taught how both methods can be valid, and that because travel is easy today, we can learn from each other as never before.

A doctor in Afghanistan taught me that a way to establish contact and reassure a patient is to clasp their ankles or wrists, and hold them firmly for a few minutes. He also showed me how to stroke softly down the body from the forehead to the feet, to produce a state of total relaxation. An Indian midwife taught me how to make deep, upward strokes on a mother's abdomen after childbirth. Among other techniques, I found it particularly useful to learn Indian head massage, which quickly refreshes and revivifies the most jaded of travelers.

❝ In India, massage is often exchanged between children and grandparents, and it is traditional to massage babies. ❞

In Sarawak, I was shown how kneading can be slow and sensuous, confirming my belief that all the main techniques can, like notes on a piano, be played with and altered, and therefore become infinitely adaptable. I also learned when not to touch at all, but to use instead flowing, mesmeric strokes just above the body, moving the air with the action and warmth of the hands, so that the recipient feels that the air itself is stroking them.

My Japanese shiatsu teacher taught me the value of applying slow, deep, and sustained pressures with one thumb on top of the other, while keeping my body totally relaxed. A Chinese teacher taught me the value of applying pressure while agitating an area, both to work an acupuncture point and to release muscular tension. In Morocco and Turkey, I learned that a thorough, effective massage is possible in as little as 15 minutes, providing enough energy and vigor is put in to almost force the muscles, and therefore the mind, to let go.

Through experiencing local massage wherever I went, I learned that all over the world the instinct to touch, to rub a sore spot to make it better, had been developed into a particular system, a body of knowledge and an art.

6 Culture by culture, "rubbing" has grown into a practice like no other, with its own silent language and vocabulary of strokes and pressures. 9

The cross-fertilization and overlap between different practices fascinated me. Even Swedish massage, which we consider to be Western, may originally have been influenced by massage from China, then systematized within the Western concept of anatomy and physiology. Many of the very gentle movements now popular in the West are also influenced by the East.

In any massage, of course, the movements must be adapted to the situation. You can massage quickly or slowly; use a light, gentle touch or a deep, strong pressure. There are only so many manipulations a hand can make, but even so, the diversity is astonishing. At one moment, you can use your hands to soothe, to calm anxiety, and to send your massage partner to sleep, and at another, you can use your hands to briskly stimulate the circulation, banish fatigue, and wake someone up feeling refreshed and ready to run a marathon! A popular expression in Thailand captures this essence: "Same, same but different."

Modern research is now confirming the power of massage. This objective proof is welcome, even essential, but it is also humbling to realize that what scientific method now substantiates has been known and tested by observation and experience throughout human history and all over the world.

In this book, I have tried to integrate many of the wonderful techniques that I have discovered over the years. They are based around the knowledge of the many different people who taught me their skills, which I have since adapted, and which are illustrated on the following pages. My hope is that this knowledge will now find a place in your own hands, hearts, and minds, and will travel further. May it be as fulfilling for you as it has been for me.

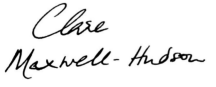

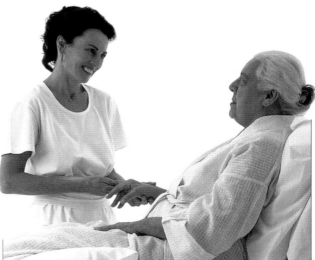

PREPARING TO MASSAGE

REGARDLESS OF THE TYPE OF MASSAGE YOU DO, there are certain principles that always apply. Try to create a peaceful sanctuary: shut the door, take the telephone off the hook, and dim the lights. Make sure that the room is warm and airy, and arrange the area so that you have enough space to move around easily. If you are cramped, it is hard to give a good massage.

YOUR PARTNER'S COMFORT

Your massage partner can lie on any firm surface. Some people prefer to lie flat, while others may need to be supported with towels or small pillows. Beds are not ideal, since they absorb the pressure of the massage in the mattress; a futon on the floor, however, is fine, or use a massage couch. Some sequences are best performed with your partner seated. Whatever the position, ensure that your partner is comfortable.

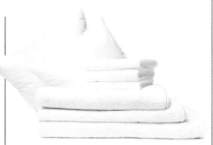

WARMTH & SUPPORT
Make sure that you have plenty of towels and small pillows to provide comfort.

PROVIDING WARMTH

Even the best massage in the world is ruined if your partner feels cold. It is virtually impossible to relax if you are chilly, so make sure that the room is warm and that you have plenty of towels. If you are working on the floor, pad the area well with a futon, a yoga mat, or several blankets so that your partner is not subjected to drafts. Remember that it is easy to become cold when lying still for a length of time, and ensure that your partner feels warm and cosseted throughout the massage. Bear in mind also that some people feel vulnerable when lying down to have a massage, so keep your partner covered with towels, and only expose the areas that you are working on. If possible, use heated towels, as

LYING FACE UP
A small pillow under the knees relaxes the muscles in the lower back, abdomen, and legs, while a folded towel under the head keeps the spine in a straight position. Spend a few minutes experimenting with the positioning of the padding, to ensure the recipient's comfort throughout the massage.

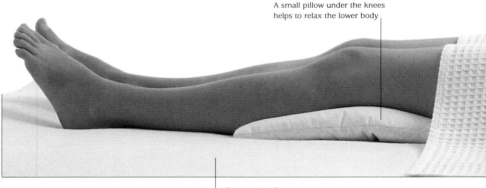

A small pillow under the knees helps to relax the lower body

A futon on the floor is an ideal massage surface

Padding under the ankles relaxes the legs

LYING FACE DOWN
A pillow or a rolled-up towel under the ankles may be comfortable for your partner, especially if she is prone to sore knees. If she has a hollow back, she may appreciate a pillow placed under the abdomen. Padding under the chest helps to release the neck area. A pillow under one shoulder also makes a useful support for some people.

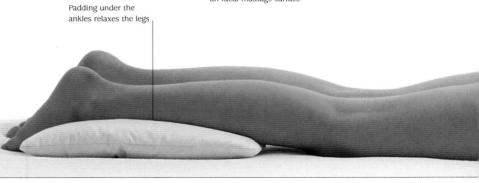

STAYING RELAXED

Whatever position you are working in, ensure that you are comfortable. Keep your back straight and use your body weight to apply pressure.

these add a touch of luxury and can help to make your partner feel pampered. In winter, or if the room is particularly cold, use a small hot-water bottle or an electric heated pad to provide extra warmth.

YOUR COMFORT

You will obviously think about your partner's position, but in order to massage successfully, your comfort is equally important. If you are comfortable, you can concentrate on your partner, whereas if you have odd aches and pains, you are more liable to focus on yourself.

Good posture is essential to avoid fatigue and backache. Make sure that your partner is close enough for you not to have to stretch to reach the body, and always face the area you are working on. Your weight should be evenly distributed: shift from one knee to the other if you are working on the floor, and from one foot to the other if you are standing. Keep your back as straight as possible and use your body weight to apply depth and pressure; brute force will only tire you and will hurt your partner. Using your body correctly will help the massage to flow.

RELAXATION & BREATHING

I believe that giving a massage can be as beneficial as receiving one. Contrary to popular belief, you do not have to get tired when massaging, and if you use your body weight correctly, the massage will leave you feeling refreshed.

I think of massage as active meditation: even if you are feeling stressed or rushed, once you start to give a massage, these irritations fall away. The soothing, hypnotic strokes not only calm your partner but also leave you feeling refreshed and energized. The more relaxed you are, the better the massage will feel. Center yourself and focus on your partner. Make a conscious effort to breathe slowly and deeply throughout the massage. It is not uncommon for a person to hold their breath when they are trying to concentrate, and I frequently have to remind new students to breathe properly when they learn to massage.

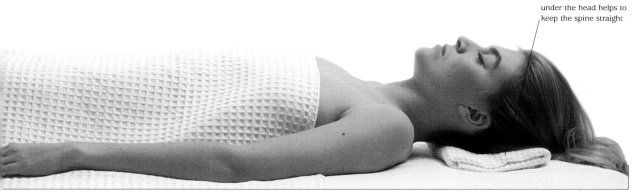

A small, folded towel under the head helps to keep the spine straight

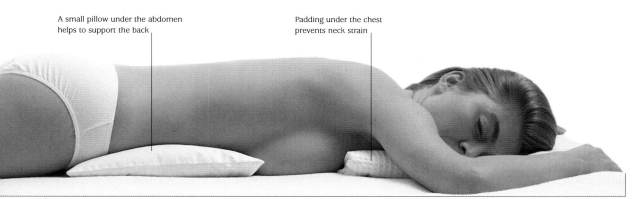

A small pillow under the abdomen helps to support the back

Padding under the chest prevents neck strain

LEARNING TO MASSAGE

THE SECRET OF A GOOD MASSAGE lies in the combination of rhythm, pressure, continuity, and focused contact. A massage should be like music, with one stroke flowing into the next. It is often the simplest of movements that feels best, so never worry if you cannot remember what to do next, just keep stroking. Repeating a movement will help you to establish the rhythm of the massage, and it is this rhythm and repetition that is so relaxing, the hands almost hypnotizing the mind and body into letting go.

THE MIND BEHIND THE MASSAGE

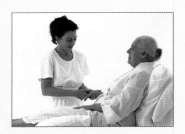

When you massage, your state of mind is just as important as your hands, and you must be relaxed and focused. The following guidelines will help you.

Take the time to tune into your partner's needs before you begin. Look at how she walks, sits, or lies, and try to see how her body responds to physical and mental stress. Which muscles does she habitually use? Does she guard herself in any way?

✦

Ask yourself what you hope to accomplish and how you can make your partner feel better. Touching with the intent to heal can produce a transfer of energy that your partner will sense. Healing is a two-way process, so make sure that your partner feels involved.

✦

Make positive statements, not negative ones, during a massage. If you notice a tense area, try to dispel the tension with your hands rather than comment on it.

✦

Silently rehearse the massage in your mind before you begin. This is one of the best ways to learn movements and sequences.

LEARNING THE TECHNIQUES

Mastering a few strokes at a time is the easiest way to learn massage. It is better to repeat the same movement, and do it really well, than to jump from one stroke to the next. In general, most movements should be repeated at least three times, but if your partner enjoys a movement and you like performing it, then keep repeating it. Always experiment with the movements and try to develop your own unique style.

ESTABLISHING A TEMPO

Match your movements to your partner's needs. If your partner feels hyperactive, begin energetically and gradually work more softly and slowly. If your partner feels lethargic, start slowly and gently, then increase the pressure and speed. Generally, slow, gentle strokes soothe, while fast, energetic strokes stimulate. If your partner falls asleep, carry on massaging; such a state of relaxation allows you to get more easily into the muscles as you stroke and knead.

APPLYING PRESSURE

There have always been differences of opinion on how much pressure to apply. The 19th-century French surgeon, Lucas Championniere, said that pressure should be "little more than a caress." Conversely, Dr. J. B. Zabludowski, a German contemporary of Championniere, stated that "massage which becomes painless ceases to be massage."

I believe that you should tailor the pressure to suit your partner. You need to apply enough pressure for it to be effective without causing pain. This varies according to the individual. Generally, pressure should be light at first, becoming deeper as the massage progresses, then gentle toward the end. To apply deep pressure, lean your body weight very slowly into the area; the smaller the point of contact, the deeper the penetration. Hold the pressure for between five and thirty seconds before releasing equally slowly. Your partner may experience slight pain, but this should be "grateful" pain, rather than "ouch" pain! Always ask for feedback on how much pressure to apply.

When giving a massage, it is common to come across areas that are painful yet seem to want to be pressed. These are the areas that we tend to press on ourselves to relieve aches and pains. They are referred to as "trigger points," "acupuncture points," "shiatsu points," "nerve motor points," or "connective tissue micro-adhesions." If a point is particularly painful, however, digging away at it may lead to muscle guarding, when the muscles tense up even more. In this case, lessen the pressure and gently stroke and stretch the area to relax it before going deeper.

DEALING WITH TICKLISHNESS

Ticklishness often indicates tension. If your massage partner is ticklish in an area, spend time stroking it. Fast finger movements can tickle, so flatten your hand, reduce the tempo, and increase the depth. If ticklishness continues, ask your partner to massage the area, or leave it until the next massage.

HAND EXERCISES

Y OUR HANDS ARE YOUR MASSAGE TOOLS and need
to be strong, flexible, relaxed, and sensitive.
Hand exercises help you to achieve this. According to
researchers at the University of Cologne in Germany,
hand exercises boost the circulation and this can also
help to keep your brain fit and enhance your memory.
When massaging, keep your wrists and hands as
relaxed as possible. If you give a massage with tense
hands, they feel hard and unfeeling, whereas a massage
with relaxed hands transmits care and support.

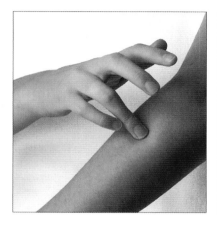

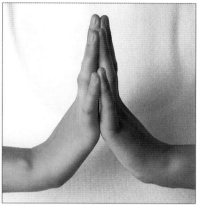

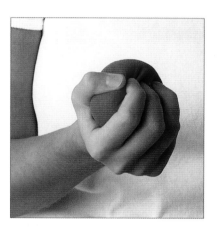

1 Drum your fingers up and down your
forearm to improve their strength and
flexibility. Vary the depth and speed of the
movement, and try not to tense your hands.
Continue for about 30 seconds.

2 For greater strength and flexibility, place
your hands together in a praying position,
then lift your elbows up so that your palms
separate. Press your fingers against each other
and hold for 10 seconds.

3 Strengthen your hands by holding a small
rubber ball in one hand, and repeatedly
squeeze and relax your fingers. Continue for
about 30 seconds, then repeat the exercise
with the other hand.

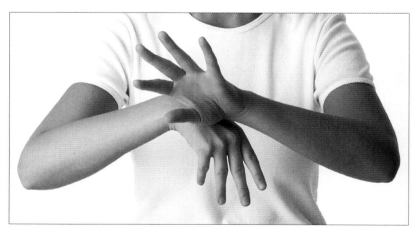

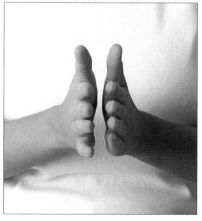

4 Improve your flexibility by placing one
wrist on the other, with your elbows
out. Roll your hands around one another
in a large circle, stretching your fingertips.
Continue for 10 seconds.

5 To increase sensitivity, hold your hands
as close as possible without touching.
Slowly draw them apart, then bring them
toward each other. Continue for a minute.
They may feel warm or begin to tingle.

CHOOSING & BLENDING OILS

USING OIL IN MASSAGE HELPS YOUR HANDS to glide over the skin and enhances the beneficial effects of the treatment. Use one of the carrier oils described below, either on its own, or scented with aromatic and therapeutic essential oils. Extracted from plants, essential oils are highly concentrated, so they must be diluted in a carrier oil before being applied to the skin.

CARRIER OILS

These oils can be used on their own, or enriched with essential oils for an aromatherapy massage.

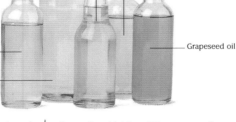

Soya oil

Sweet almond oil

Apricot kernel oil

Sunflower oil

Grapeseed oil

CARRIER OILS

Rich in vitamins, proteins, and minerals, carrier oils help to moisturize the skin and keep it supple. Some of the most commonly used carrier oils are sweet almond oil, apricot kernel oil, sunflower oil, soya oil, and grapeseed oil. Try to choose cold-pressed oils, which are generally of better quality than heat- or solvent-extracted oils. To enrich the moisturizing and nourishing properties of an oil, add 10 to 20 percent of a special carrier oil, such as avocado oil, sesame oil, wheat germ oil, or jojoba oil.

OIL BLENDS

Before blending, decide if you are going to use oils on their own, to pamper and moisturize the skin, or if you wish to blend in essential oils that will stimulate or calm the recipient (*see table, opposite*). If you decide to use essential oils, it is very important that you use a safe dilution, or the oil may irritate the skin. Oil blends are generally referred to as normal or low dilutions, based on the percentage of essential oil in the carrier oil. A normal dilution is 2 percent and a low dilution is 1 percent. To calculate how many drops of essential oil you need for each dilution, see the blending guide below. There is no need to include more than two or three oils in a blend. For a full-body massage, you will need about 4 tsp (20ml) of oil; for a face massage, you will need about 2 tsp (10ml).

GUIDE TO BLENDING OILS

Normal dilution of 2 percent
For every 2 tsp (10ml) carrier oil you blend, add up to 4 drops essential oil.

✦

Low dilution of 1 percent
For every 2 tsp (10ml) carrier oil you blend, add up to 2 drops essential oil.

✦

Extremely low dilution of 0.5 percent, for children, babies, and sensitive skins
For every 2 tsp (10ml) carrier oil you blend, add 1 drop essential oil. Alternatively, you can massage with carrier oil alone.

MAKING AN OIL BLEND

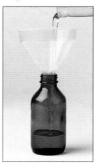

1 To make an oil blend, decant the amount of carrier oil that you need into a dark glass bottle. Choose two or three essential oils (*see opposite*), and add the appropriate number of drops for the required dilution into the carrier oil.

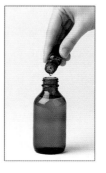

2 Close the bottle, shake it well, and label it clearly, noting the oils used, the dilution, and the date. In general, essential oil blends should be used within a few weeks.

ESSENTIAL OILS

When using essential oils, try to choose a blend that appeals to your partner. Scents can be divided into notes: top notes are the first impressions of a scent, middle notes are the body of the scent, and base notes are released last. Combining all three notes generally ensures a well-rounded perfume. The chart below lists some of my favorite essential oils. The common name of each oil is followed by the botanical name of the plant from which it derives. The scent's main characteristics and predominant notes are also given.

GUIDE TO ESSENTIAL OILS

ESSENTIAL OIL	SCENT	SCENT NOTE	THERAPEUTIC PROPERTIES	CAUTIONS
FRANKINCENSE *Boswellia carterii*	Balsamic, rich, sweet	Middle/Base	Calming, mucus reductional, used to combat the ageing process	
YLANG YLANG *Cananga odorata*	Heady, floral, exotic	Middle/Base	Anti-depressant, sedative, euphoric	Use in low dilutions
ROMAN CHAMOMILE *Chamaemelum nobile*	Pungent, herbaceous	Top/Middle	Calming, anti-spasmodic, suitable for sensitive skins	
NEROLI *Citrus aurantium*	Orange blossom, light, sweet, floral	Top/Middle	Gently sedative, anti-depressant, used for emotional problems	Use in low dilutions, avoid sun after use
ORANGE *Citrus aurantium*	Orange fruit, fresh, citrus-like, dry	Top	Uplifting, anti-spasmodic, mildly astringent	Avoid sun for 6 hours after use (*see opposite*)
CYPRESS *Cupressus sempervirens*	Spicy, sweet, refreshing	Top/Middle	Anti-spasmodic, used for respiratory problems, astringent, anti-rheumatic	Avoid in first 3 months of pregnancy
EUCALYPTUS *Eucalyptus globulus*	Camphor-like, sweet, woody	Top	Antiseptic, eases pains, stimulating, used for respiratory complaints	Use in low dilutions
JASMINE *Jasminum officinale*	Sweet, heady, floral	Top/Middle/Base	Uplifting, anti-depressant, used to treat lethargy, invigorating	Avoid in pregnancy and on babies
JUNIPER *Juniperus communis*	Woody, fresh, sweet	Top	Eases aches and pains, antiseptic, anti-rheumatic, diuretic	Avoid in pregnancy
LAVENDER *Lavandula angustifolia*	Piercing, sweet, floral	Middle	Sedative, antiseptic, analgesic	
GERMAN CHAMOMILE *Matricaria recutita*	Pungent, herbaceous	Top/Middle	Anti-inflammatory, soothing, suitable for sensitive skins	
PEPPERMINT *Mentha piperita*	Minty, fresh, grass-like	Top	Stimulating, eases headaches, anti-spasmodic action on the gut	Use in low dilutions
GERANIUM *Pelargonium graveolens*	Sweet, floral, herbaceous	Top/Middle	Anti-depressant, anti-bacterial, astringent	Use in low dilutions
ROSE *Rosa x centifolia/R. x damascena*	Intense, floral	Top/Middle/Base	Anti-depressant, antiseptic, calming	
ROSEMARY *Rosmarinus officinalis*	Piercing, fresh, herbaceous	Top/Middle	Stimulating, eases aches, clears congestion	Avoid in pregnancy, high blood pressure, epilepsy
CLARY SAGE *Salvia sclarea*	Warm, nutty, herbaceous	Top	Anti-depressant, warming, anti-spasmodic tonic	Avoid in pregnancy and with alcohol
SANDALWOOD *Santalum album*	Sweet, woody, balsamic	Base	Calming, antiseptic, used to treat problem skins	
GINGER *Zingiber officinale*	Spicy, camphor-like	Middle/Base	Warming, stimulating	Use in low dilutions

THE POWER OF MASSAGE

MASSAGE PROVIDES A POSITIVE WAY to demonstrate care and concern, and can have profound effects on health and well-being. It helps to promote mental and physical relaxation, its therapeutic benefits can ease a wide range of ailments, and a physiologically stimulating massage can have a psychologically relaxing effect. Research is now verifying the many therapeutic claims that have been made for massage.

AN AID TO HEALING

Massage has been found to be helpful in the treatment of a variety of conditions, including stress-related ailments such as tension headaches, insomnia, high blood pressure, and backache. It can relieve depression, anxiety, and pain. It can also alleviate musculo-skeletal problems, such as arthritis and back pain, and digestive disorders such as constipation and stress-related abdominal pain.

It is not, however, only the recipient who benefits from a massage. I maintain that there are physical and psychological benefits for both the giver and the receiver, and they can emerge from a massage equally refreshed and relaxed.

KEY BENEFITS

Massage has a positive effect on the body's physiological and psychological functions. It can help with the following:

Stimulating the circulation and speeding up the elimination of waste products.

✦

Easing sore or tense muscles.

✦

Improving flexibility.

✦

Facilitating general body relaxation.

✦

Improving wellbeing.

✦

Easing psychological tensions.

✦

Enhancing body awareness.

✦

Promoting regular sleep patterns.

PRECAUTIONS

Although massage is generally of enormous benefit, there are a few occasions when you should avoid it. If you are ever in doubt about whether to massage an area, avoid it, even if you long to help. Contraindications are unique to the individual, but in general you should never massage someone with the following conditions without obtaining the advice of their doctor:

✦ *Any serious medical condition.*
✦ *A high temperature.*
✦ *An infection or contagious disease.*

Take care in the case of any of the following conditions. Avoid the "local" conditions listed, and massage an alternative, unaffected area instead.

✦ *Edema, acute inflammation, or bruising.*
✦ *An open wound, recent scar tissue, skin infection, weeping skin condition, broken skin, or rash.*
✦ *Acute back pain, especially if the pain shoots down the legs or arms when you massage the back or neck.*
✦ *Undiagnosed lumps.*

✦ *Varicose veins, phlebitis, or thrombosis. Thrombosis can be difficult to recognize, as symptoms may vary considerably. Show caution if there is vague aching in one leg, and refer the person to their doctor.*
✦ *If your partner is pregnant, massage the abdomen and lower back very gently during the first three months.*
✦ *If someone suffers from chronic fatigue, keep your movements gentle.*
✦ *In cases of osteoporosis or joint pain, take care, and keep your massage gentle, avoiding any deep massage work.*

A MASSAGE SEQUENCE

Although each massage is different, there is often a pattern to the sequence of movements. After a hold to introduce the masseur's touch, a massage tends to start with gentle, soothing strokes. Deeper movements, such as kneading and pressures, are then gradually introduced, interspersed with stroking. The length of the massage and how you finish it depend on the effect you wish to achieve. I allow about an hour for a full-body massage.

> ## APPLYING OIL
>
> *Never pour oil directly on to the skin; warm 1 tsp (5ml) oil in your palms first. If you need more oil, drizzle it on the back of one hand and stroke it on with the other.*

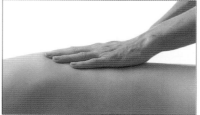

1 HOLDS Use a simple, positive hold to begin a massage. This makes initial contact with your massage partner, and says hello with your hands.

2 APPLYING THE OIL Apply the oil with light strokes, keeping the hands relaxed. When you need more oil, apply it as directed above, so contact with the body is not lost.

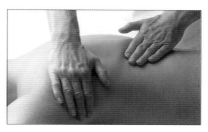

3 DEEPER STROKES Gradually increase the depth of the stroking. Mold your hands around the contours of the body, both to soothe and to feel for any tension.

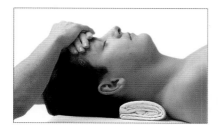

4 KNEADING Knead the area to warm it. This deeper movement will also stretch the tissue, and relieve muscle tightness and congestion.

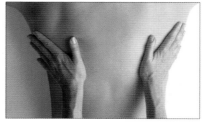

5 LINKING STROKES Stroke the body again, both as a linking movement and to relax the area and encourage the elimination of waste products.

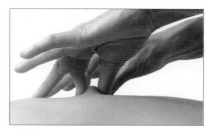

6 STRONGER MOVEMENTS Now that the area is relaxed, introduce deeper movements such as raking, knuckle strokes, circular pressures, or skin rolling.

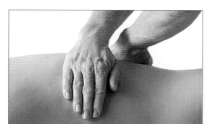

7 STROKES Relax the body after deep massage work by rhythmically stroking your hands over the whole area. Use the strokes to connect the different parts of the body with each other.

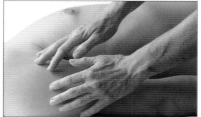

8 FEATHER STROKING Use very light, superficial feather strokes with your fingertips. These will lift away the last vestiges of tension, and let your partner know that the massage is nearly complete.

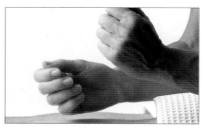

9 PERCUSSION Say goodbye, either by using brisk, stimulating percussion movements to wake your partner up, or by finishing the massage as you started, and using calm, positive holds.

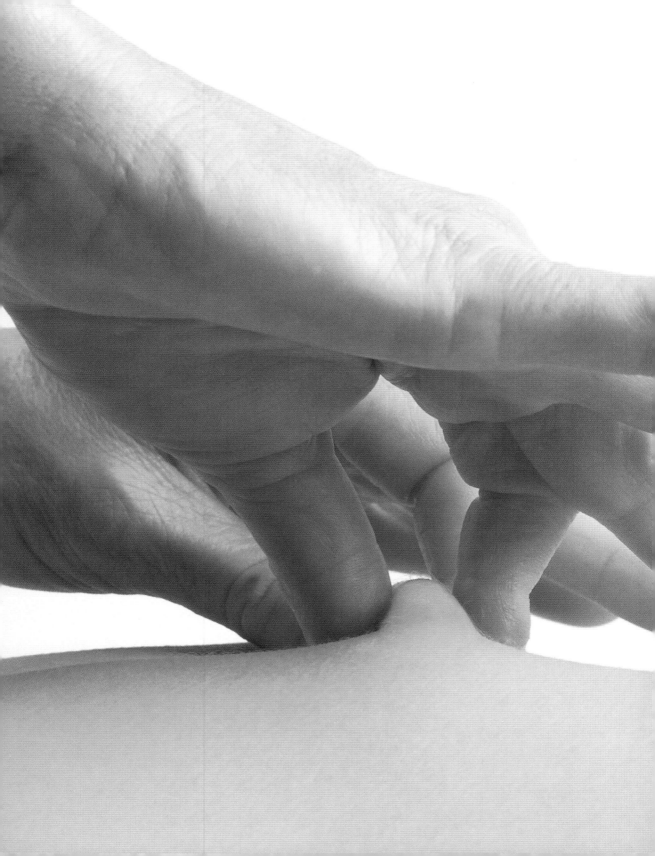

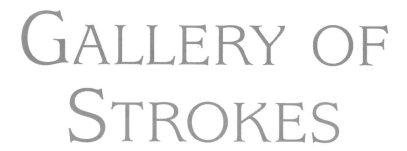

GALLERY OF STROKES

THE WORDLESS COMMUNICATION BETWEEN THE HAND THAT

GIVES THE MASSAGE AND THE BODY THAT RECEIVES IT IS

EXTRAORDINARILY PRECISE. THE MOVEMENTS RANGE FROM

THE LIGHTEST BRUSH IN THE AIR ABOVE THE SKIN TO DEEPLY

MODULATED PRESSURES AND SWEEPS; FROM MOVEMENTS

THAT ROCK THE BODY TO THOSE THAT ROLL THE MUSCLES.

THE INDIVIDUAL STROKES ARE THE BASIC COMPONENTS

OF A MASSAGE THAT CAN BE VARIED ALMOST INFINITELY

AND BLENDED TO MAKE YOUR OWN UNIQUE STYLE.

KEY TO SYMBOLS

LEVEL ★ Easy ★★ Intermediate ★★★ Difficult
OIL (*see pages 14–15*) ✓ Advised ✗ Not advised

STROKING

STROKING IS THE MOST VERSATILE OF ALL MASSAGE TECHNIQUES. It allows you to get a feel for your partner's body at the start of a massage and serves as a useful link between other movements. You can give a complete body massage with stroking alone, simply by varying the pressure and tempo of the movements. Light, superficial strokes have a soothing, hypnotic effect, while deeper ones compress the muscle tissue against the bone and stimulate the circulation. In general, you should increase pressure as you stroke toward the heart, and reduce it as you glide away from it. Try to visualize flowing water as you stroke, and replicate its effortless fluidity in your movements.

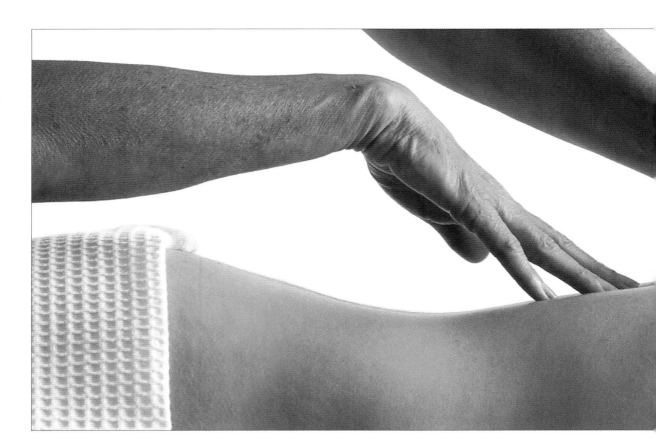

LIGHT STROKING

Gentle strokes with the whole hand or just the fingertips affect the nerve endings in the skin and have a calming influence throughout the body. They are generally used at the beginning or end of a massage, and range from sweeping the hands softly and rhythmically over the surface of the skin to aura stroking, when you do not touch the body at all.

CAT STROKING

This simple stroke can be used to apply oil at the beginning of a massage or as a final soothing touch at the end. Place one hand at the top of the area you are massaging and stroke gently down the body, molding your palm and fingers to its contours. Lift your hand off at the bottom of the area and return it to the start while your other hand begins the downward stroke. Continue, stroking one hand after the other and making the return movement as smooth and rhythmic as the stroke itself. Repeat for as long as you like – the sheer repetitiveness is what is so relaxing.

CAT STROKING
BEST FOR *Back*   LEVEL ★   OIL ✓   EFFECT *Calms the nerves; soporific*

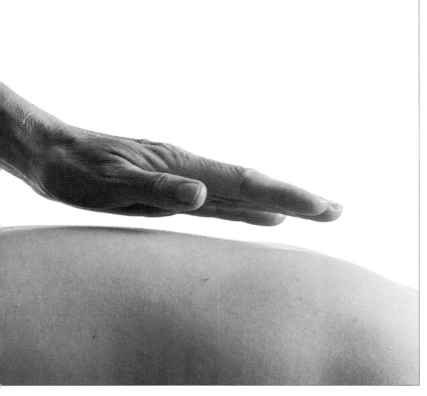

FEATHER STROKING

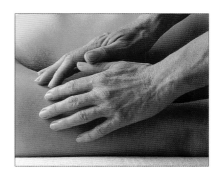

Sometimes known as nerve stroking, this movement can induce deep relaxation. Stroke the fingertips of both your hands very lightly down the body. Repeat, and as you continue, stroke more and more gently until you are barely touching the skin at all. Most people love this superficial stroke, but some may find it too ticklish.

FEATHER STROKING
BEST FOR *Whole body*   LEVEL ★   OIL ✓
EFFECT *Soothing, sedative*

AURA STROKING

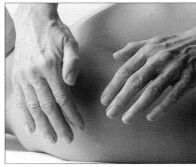

Place your hands side by side just above the surface of the skin and slowly move them together over the area. As your hands begin to generate heat, your partner may feel a warm, tingling sensation. Aura stroking is used by practitioners, particularly in traditional cultures such as India, China, and Afghanistan, to disperse "blockages" in a person's "field of energy."

AURA STROKING
BEST FOR *Back, abdomen, legs, arms*
LEVEL ★   OIL ✗
EFFECT *Creates warm, tingling feeling; relaxing*

Fan Stroking

The secret of this fluid movement
is to mold your hands to the curves
of the body without dragging the skin,
and to maintain a steady rhythm. The
length of the strokes can vary, but your
hands should never lose contact with the
skin. Alternate fan stroking (*see pages 24–25*)
is a slight variation, creating soothing
diagonal stretches. For a deeper, more
precise action, the thumbs can be used
in a fanning movement.

Fan Stroking on the Back

1 Place your palms side by side on the lower back on
either side of the spine. Stroke up the back, applying
a firm pressure with the palms of your hands.

2 When you reach the top of the back, open your
fingers and fan your hands out away from the
spine, reducing the pressure as you do so.

3 Now glide your hands down the sides of the body,
molding your palms and fingers to its contours.
Apply less pressure on this downward stroke.

4 Pull up slightly at the waist and return your hands
to the starting position. Repeat the movement
several times to achieve fluidity, varying the length of
the upward stroke each time to cover the whole back.

Fan Stroking

Best for *Large areas, such as the back*
Level ★ Oil ✓
Effect *Soothing*

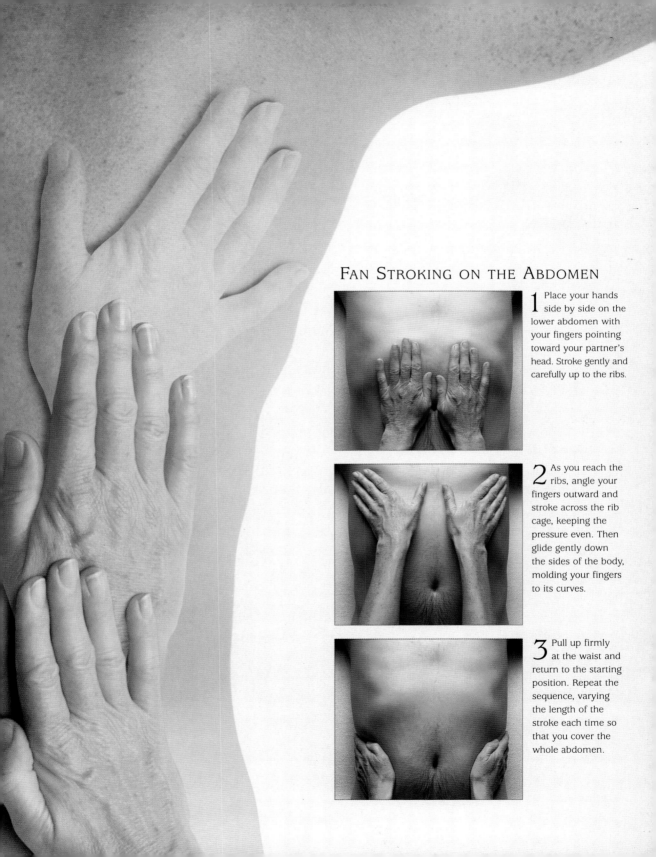

FAN STROKING ON THE ABDOMEN

1 Place your hands side by side on the lower abdomen with your fingers pointing toward your partner's head. Stroke gently and carefully up to the ribs.

2 As you reach the ribs, angle your fingers outward and stroke across the rib cage, keeping the pressure even. Then glide gently down the sides of the body, molding your fingers to its curves.

3 Pull up firmly at the waist and return to the starting position. Repeat the sequence, varying the length of the stroke each time so that you cover the whole abdomen.

ALTERNATE FAN STROKING

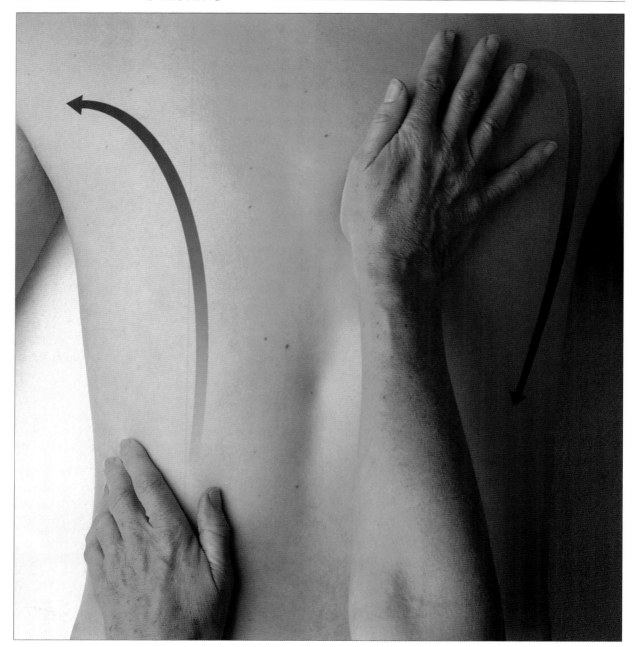

1 For this variation on the simple fan stroke, place both your hands side by side, as you would begin for fan stroking (*see pages 22–23*). Stroke your right hand up the body, keeping the pressure firm and even, and as you reach the top of the area, fan your fingers out towards the side, molding them around the body's contours.

2 ▲ Glide your right hand down the side of the body as your left hand starts the movement, fanning out to the left. Repeat, so that as one hand strokes firmly up the body, the other glides down. Try to keep the strokes as flowing as possible, and with practice, this should become a wonderfully smooth and rhythmic stroke.

ALTERNATE FAN STROKING

BEST FOR *Back, legs, arms*
LEVEL ★★   OIL ✓
EFFECT *Creates soothing diagonal stretches*

FAN STROKING WITH THUMBS

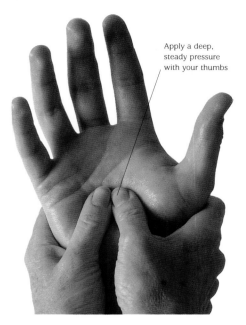

Apply a deep, steady pressure with your thumbs

1 Supporting the part of the body you are working on with your fingers, stroke both thumbs firmly up the area as far as you can reach.

2 At the top of the area, reduce the pressure and stroke your thumbs out to the sides. Glide lightly back around to the starting position and repeat the sequence several times.

Stroke out to the sides of the area

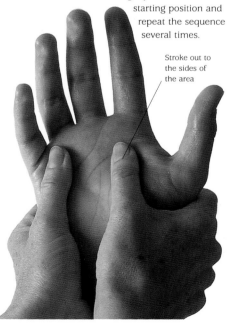

ALTERNATE FAN STROKING WITH THUMBS

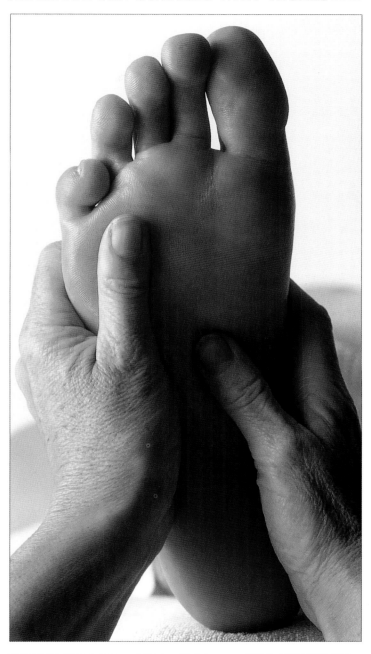

Support the area you are working on with the fingers of both hands, and stroke one thumb firmly upward and out to the side. As you reach the top of the area, follow with your other thumb and return your first thumb to the starting position. Repeat several times, trying to stroke higher up the area each time.

FAN & ALTERNATE FAN STROKING WITH THUMBS

BEST FOR *Hands, feet, forehead*
LEVEL ★   OIL ✓
EFFECT *Eases away tension*

CIRCLE STROKING

Circle stroking is a flowing, continuous movement that can be used to spread oil around the body and to link movements in a complete massage. The direction in which you stroke is up to you, although on the stomach you should stroke in a clockwise direction to follow the workings of the intestines. Light, circular strokes with the fingertips skim over the skin, creating a soft, soothing effect. Deep, slow circle stroking uses your body weight and molds the flesh. It can be used on the back, shoulders, and backs of the thighs, and is an effective way to help stretch tight muscles. To ease tension in small, tight areas, circle with the thumbs.

LIGHT CIRCLE STROKING

1 Place your hands apart on the body, with your fingers pointing forward. Start to stroke your left hand gently in a large circle, either in a clockwise or counterclockwise direction. Stroke the right hand in the same way.

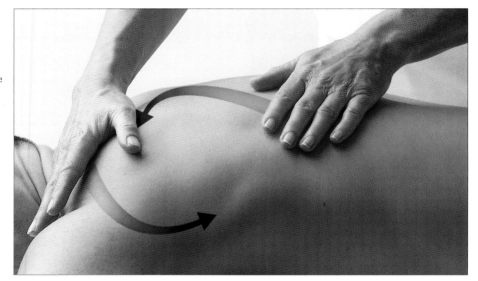

2 As one hand meets the other wrist, lift it over, and place it lightly on the other side to complete the circle, as the other hand continues stroking. Repeat the sequence, applying slightly more pressure on the upward and outward stroke, and reducing the pressure as you glide down and in. Try to build up a steady rhythm.

**LIGHT & DEEP
CIRCLE STROKING**

BEST FOR *Shoulders, abdomen, hips*
LEVEL ★★   OIL ✓
EFFECT *Soothes if light; stretches if deep*

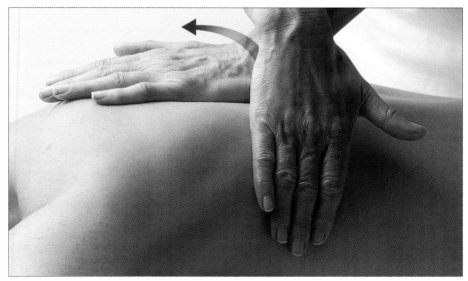

DEEP CIRCLE STROKING

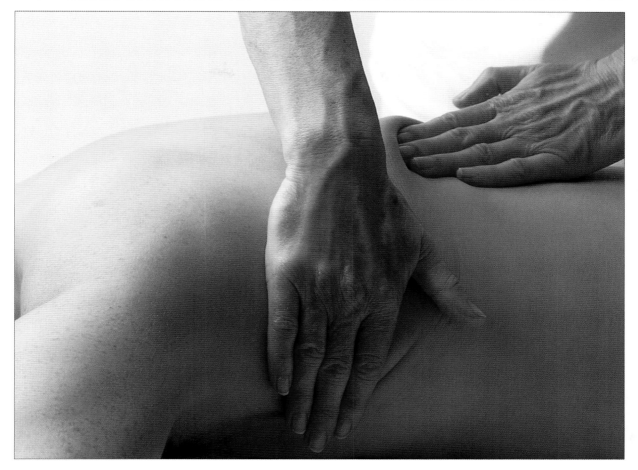

For deep circle stroking, follow the sequence for Light Circle Stroking (*see opposite*) but as you stroke, lean into the movement with your body weight and use the fingers and heels of your hands to mold and sculpt the flesh. If you are working on the back, make sure that you do not press on the spine.

CIRCULAR THUMB STROKING

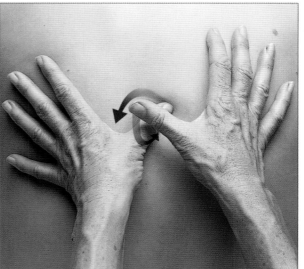

1 Place both hands on the body, with your thumbs slightly apart. With your fingers still resting on the body, start stroking both thumbs in a circle, one thumb following the other. Press firmly as you stroke upward and outward.

2 ▶ When one thumb meets the other, lift it over and continue the circle on the other side, releasing the pressure on the downward stroke. One thumb completes a circle while the other one does a half circle. Keep the movement precise.

CIRCULAR THUMB STROKING

BEST FOR *Small, tense areas*
LEVEL ★★   OIL ✓
EFFECT *Loosens tight, knotted areas*

SIDE STROKING

One of the most simple massage techniques to master, side stroking is extraordinarily soothing for both giver and receiver. Its repetitiveness has a hypnotic effect, and as your partner relaxes, you can apply deeper pressure. Light side stroking is performed with very relaxed hands in a flowing movement, and it affects nerve endings in the skin. It should be performed in a smooth, flowing sequence and is a useful way to ease any tension in your hands after deeper work such as kneading (*see page 34*). Deep side stroking uses the whole hand and the forearms, and works on the muscles, helping to stretch muscular tissue.

LIGHT SIDE STROKING

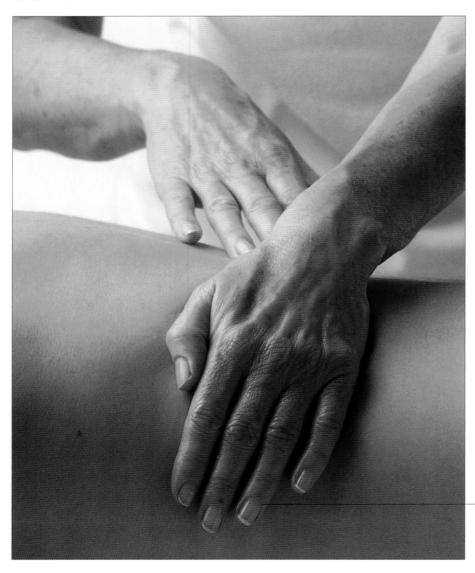

1 ◄ Face your partner's side and place both hands on the far side of the body, fingers pointing downward. Stroke your right hand lightly and slowly up the side of the body toward you, and follow with your left hand in the same way.

2 Lift your right hand away as you reach the top of the body and repeat with your left hand. Continue, so that one hand follows the other in a relaxed, continuous movement. If you are working on the side closest to you, push up with your hands or swivel yourself around so that you can pull up instead. Remember always to keep your back straight.

LIGHT SIDE STROKING

BEST FOR *Back, abdomen, thighs*
LEVEL ★   OIL ✓
EFFECT *Calms the nerves; hypnotic*

Use relaxed fingertips to stroke lightly and smoothly

DEEP SIDE STROKING

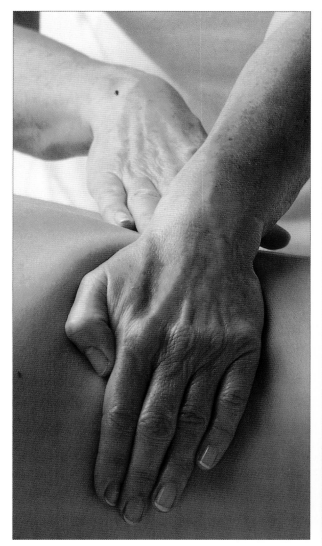

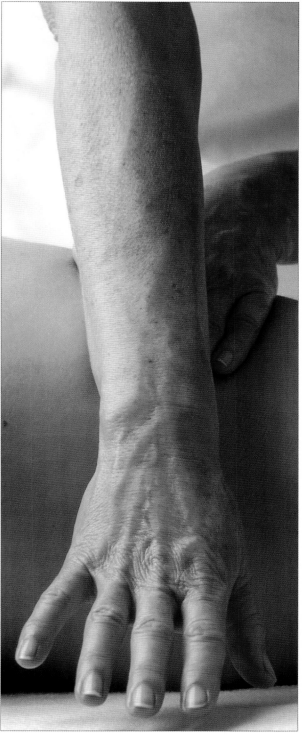

1 ▲ Face the side of your partner and place both your hands on their opposite side, with your fingers pointing away from you. Stroke one hand firmly up the side and use your body weight to make the movement deep, pulling in and up toward you, and molding the flesh with the heel and fingers of your hand.

2 ▶ When your hand reaches the top of the body, lift it off as you start the movement with your other hand. Repeat several times, gradually working more slowly and deeply, and using your forearms as well as your hands to stroke the body.

DEEP SIDE STROKING

BEST FOR *Back, abdomen, thighs*
LEVEL ★   OIL ✔
EFFECT *Releases muscular tension*

CRISS-CROSSING STROKES

Strokes that criss-cross the body combine smooth, gliding movements with gentle squeezes. Both hands work simultaneously to create a fluid rhythm that is wonderfully relaxing for the recipient. Simple criss-crosses are easy to learn and can be used all over the body, although you should avoid pressing the spine. If you are working on the legs, take care not to pinch the flesh, and do not use this technique if there are varicose veins. Figures of eight may require practice in order to achieve a smooth and seamless motion.

SIMPLE CRISS-CROSSES

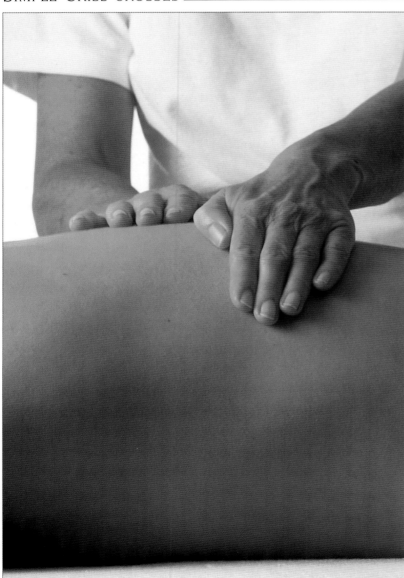

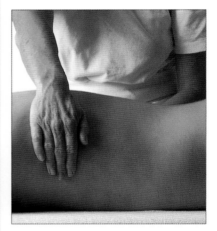

1 ◄ Face your partner's side and place one hand on each side of the area, with your fingers facing away from you. Pull one hand and push the other firmly up each side and glide them smoothly across the body.

2 Slide your hands past each other and down toward the other side of the body. Make a distinction between firmly pulling up at the sides and then very gently gliding across the skin. Repeat the stroke, working along the whole area systematically.

SIMPLE CRISS-CROSSES

BEST FOR *Back, abdomen, legs, arms*
LEVEL ★   OIL ✓
EFFECT *Soothes and comforts*

FIGURES OF EIGHT

BEST FOR *Back, thighs*
LEVEL ★★   OIL ✓
EFFECT *Induces deep relaxation*

FIGURES OF EIGHT

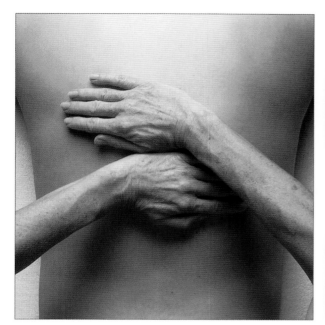

1 Place your hands side by side on the skin so that the fingers of one hand face the opposite way to the fingers of the other hand. Gently glide your hands out to the sides of the area.

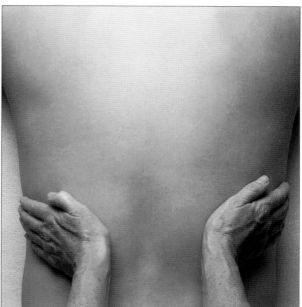

2 As you reach the edges of the area, swivel your fingers around as smoothly as possible, then pull them upward so that you gently squeeze the sides of the body.

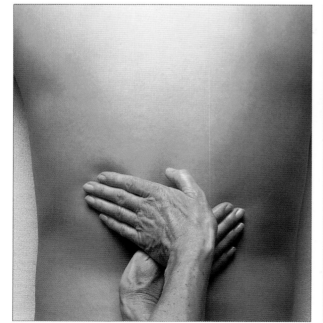

3 Reduce the pressure and glide your hands across the body again, a little further down from the point where you started. Keep the movement fluid as one hand passes the other.

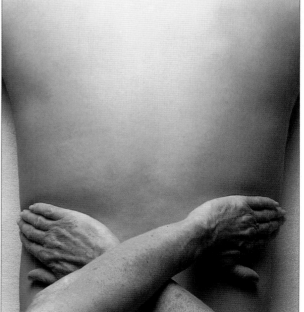

4 Swivel your fingers around so that your arms cross and pull up at the sides again. Then continue with these figures of eight down the area, working as rhythmically as you can.

DEEP STROKING

Strokes can be deep enough to compress the muscle tissue against the bone. They should only be used once an area has been sufficiently relaxed with gentle stroking and are especially effective on large muscle groups. Deep strokes have a broadening and stretching action on the muscle tissue, and should generally follow the direction of the muscle fibers. On the back, work up or down with deep strokes on the muscles, taking care to avoid the spine; on the limbs, stroke toward the torso, following the circulation.

FOREARM STROKES

Face the side of your partner and rest one hand or forearm on the body as a support. With your other forearm, stroke firmly up the area, slowly rotating your arm to give a deep pressure that lengthens and compresses the muscular tissue. Make sure that your hand is relaxed so that the pressure comes from the arm. In a Hawaiian form of massage known as *Lomi Lomi*, this forearm stroking is aptly described as "ironing". You can also stroke both your forearms in opposite directions to create more of a stretch.

FOREARM STROKES

BEST FOR *Back, thighs*
LEVEL ★★   OIL ✓
EFFECT *Irons out tension*

Slowly rotate your forearm as you stroke it up the area

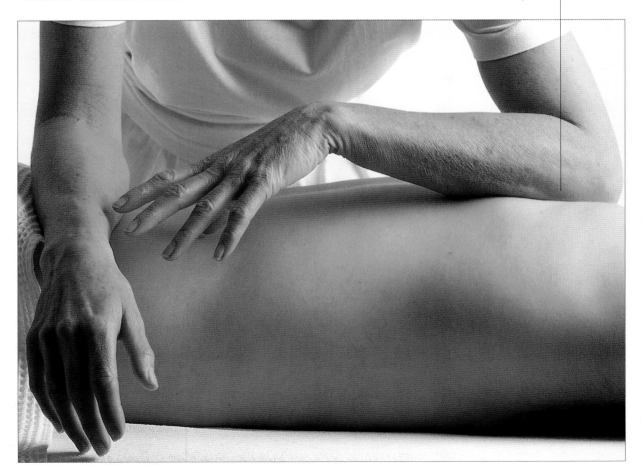

KNUCKLE STROKES

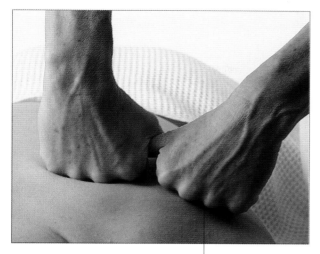

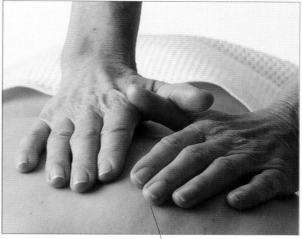

1 Loosely clench your fists, interlocking your thumbs for support, and stroke your knuckles firmly up the area, using your body weight to apply a deep pressure.

Stroke your knuckles firmly up the skin

2 Roll your fingers out from under your palms and gently stroke your hands back down the area. Then make your hands into fists again and repeat the whole movement, aiming for a wave-like motion. This stroke is particularly relaxing for the giver.

Glide your hands back down the area

KNUCKLE STROKES

BEST FOR *Either side of spine; arms*
LEVEL ★   OIL ✔
EFFECT *Eases taut muscles*

RAKING

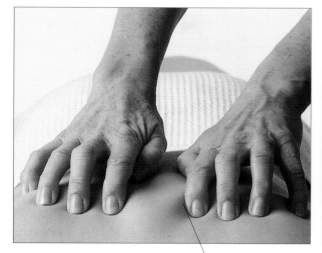

Flex the fingers of both hands so that they are quite rigid and rake-like, and stroke them toward you, either together or alternately. When you reach the end of the area, return your hands to the start and repeat.

Stroke deeply and smoothly

RAKING

BEST FOR *Back (either parallel or at right angles to spine)*
LEVEL ★   OIL ✔
EFFECT *Deeply relaxing*

V-STROKES

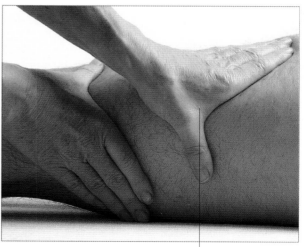

Using the V-shape between your thumb and fingers, stroke one hand after the other up the area in a firm motion, shaping your hands around the body. Keep your hands relaxed, with the depth coming from your body.

Mold your hands to the shape of the body

V-STROKES

BEST FOR *Bulky, muscular areas*
LEVEL ★★   OIL ✔
EFFECT *Warms and relaxes*

KNEADING

USED TO RELAX AND SOFTEN AN AREA, kneading involves squeezing, lifting, and rolling the flesh. It helps to create space around the muscle fibers, making them more pliable, and eases tension in the connective tissue that surrounds every muscle (*see page 161*). The success of kneading relies on an even rhythm and, as with all strokes, the depth and speed can vary. A steady tempo is generally effective, and I have found that fast kneading can be extremely stimulating whereas slow kneading has more of a soporific effect. Sometimes the muscles in your partner's body may be so tight that it is difficult to lift the skin. In this case, just knead the area with flat hands; the rhythm of the movement should relax the area enough for you to get in deeper at a later stage.

BASIC KNEADING

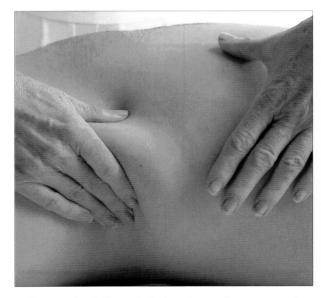

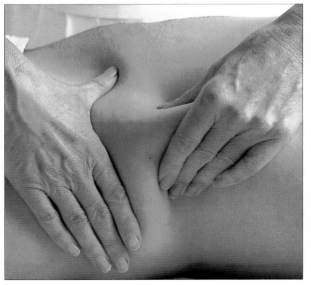

1 Place your hands flat on the body with your elbows out to each side and fingers pointing toward each other. With your right hand, gently grasp and squeeze some flesh, using as much of the hand as possible to avoid pinching the skin. Then release and push the flesh toward your left hand. If there is not much flesh to pick up, follow this movement superficially.

2 Grasp the flesh with your left hand in the same way, then release it into your right hand again. Repeat several times, pushing the flesh from side to side as if kneading bread, and counting to keep your strokes even and rhythmic.

BASIC KNEADING

BEST FOR *Fleshy areas, such as the hips or buttocks*
LEVEL ★★   OIL ✓
EFFECT *Relaxes and stretches tight muscles*

WRINGING

This is a deeper movement than basic kneading. Pull the flesh up with one hand, then twist it into your other hand, pressing into it with your thumbs. Imagine that you are wringing out a towel as you twist the flesh from one hand to the other.

WRINGING

BEST FOR *Fleshy areas, such as the hips or buttocks*
LEVEL ★★   OIL ✓   EFFECT *Loosens and stimulates*

ONE-HANDED KNEADING

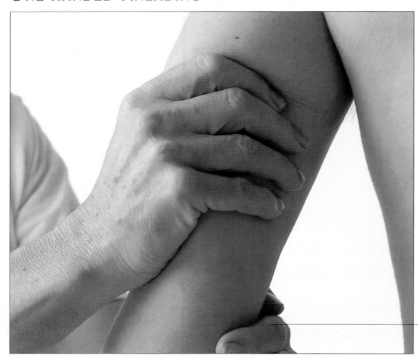

◀ **This is a useful stroke** for areas of the body where there is not enough room for two hands to work effectively. Support the area with one hand and squeeze and release the flesh with the other hand. If working on the arm, you can use alternate hands on either side to squeeze and release.

ONE-HANDED KNEADING
BEST FOR *Tops of shoulders; arms; calves*
LEVEL ★   OIL ✔
EFFECT *Softens and relaxes*

Support the area with one hand

FINGERTIP KNEADING

▶ **This movement is very small** and precise. Lift and squeeze the flesh with the thumb and fingers of one hand, then glide it toward the other hand. Repeat the movement with the thumb and fingers of the other hand. Remember to keep your elbows out as you pull the flesh up so that you avoid pinching the skin.

FINGERTIP KNEADING
BEST FOR *Areas without much flesh, such as the neck and upper arms*
LEVEL ★★   OIL ✔
EFFECT *Relaxes the skin and top layers of muscle*

Squeeze the flesh between your fingers and thumb

SKIN ROLLING

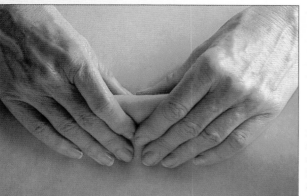

1 Place your hands on the skin so that you create a triangular shape between your fingers and thumbs. Then, without sliding your fingers on the skin, pull the flesh toward your thumbs.

2 ◄ Push your thumbs firmly toward your fingers, rolling the flesh as you do so, and taking care not to pinch the skin as your thumbs meet your fingers. Then reach forward with your fingers again and repeat the movement as rhythmically as possible.

SKIN ROLLING

BEST FOR *Shoulders, back (either parallel or at right angles to the spine)*
LEVEL ★★   OIL ✓
EFFECT *Loosens tight areas*

ALTERNATIVE METHOD

For another form of skin rolling, slide your thumbs toward your forefingers so that they squeeze the flesh, then walk your fingers forward as your thumbs push the flesh behind. I call this movement "inchworming".

Walk your fingers along the body

PRESSURES

S TATIC AND CIRCULAR PRESSURES range from deep, precise movements with the thumbs or fingers, to broader compressions with the heel of the hand: the smaller the area, the deeper the penetration. Light pressures are soothing and allow you to feel for tense muscles; deeper pressures compress tight muscle bands, and may break down adhesions. Use your body weight to achieve depth, and only apply deep pressure to previously massaged areas. Some effective common techniques are shown opposite.

STATIC & CIRCULAR PRESSURES

▶ **Static pressures** should be applied slowly and steadily. Lean into the pressure with your body weight, hold for a few seconds, then gradually release and glide to the next area. As the skin tissue relaxes and stretches, deeper pressure can be applied.

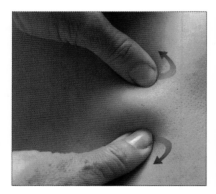

Circular pressures, sometimes known as friction, require that the hand and skin work together as one, so that you move the superficial layer of flesh against the deeper tissue in a circular motion. Experiment with fast, superficial circles and slow, deep ones. After deep pressures, always gently stroke and soothe the area.

STATIC & CIRCULAR PRESSURES

BEST FOR *Tight, knotted areas*
LEVEL ★★   OIL ✗
EFFECT *May break down any muscular adhesions*

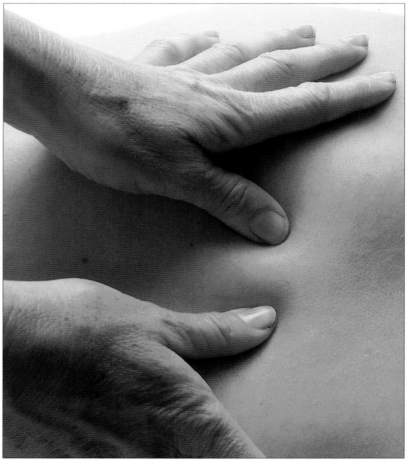

A SELECTION OF PRESSURES

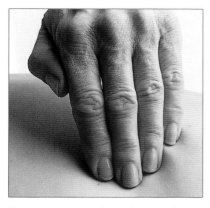

Finger pressures can be static or circular. Use three or four fingers to apply pressure while your other hand supports the area.

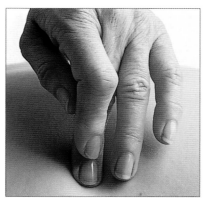

Cross your index finger over your middle finger to apply a deep, static pressure. Alternatively, agitate the fingers on the spot.

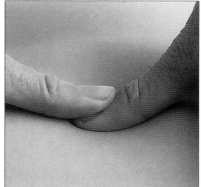

One thumb on top of the other produces a very deep pressure that is extremely effective for cross-fiber work.

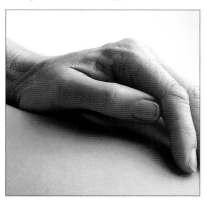

The heel of the hand creates a broad pressure that can be circular or static. Make sure that your fingers are relaxed.

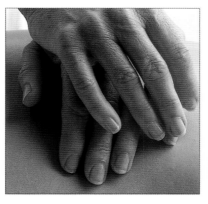

Put one hand on top of the other for a deep pressure. Lean over your hands so that the strength comes from your body.

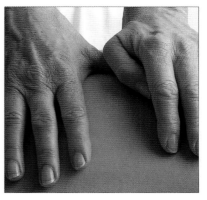

Place the heel of one hand over the thumb of the other. Keep the thumb flat, so that the pressure is deep but diffused.

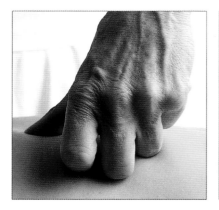

Roll your knuckles deeply into the flesh, using slow, circular movements. You can use your thumb as a support.

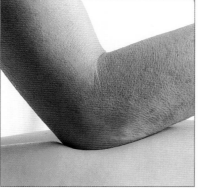

The elbow creates a particularly deep pressure. Relax your arm so that you use your body weight to ease into the flesh.

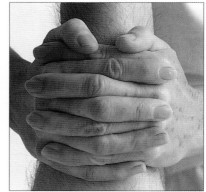

Interlock your fingers and squeeze the flesh with the palms of your hands. This pressure is often called a "compression."

PERCUSSION

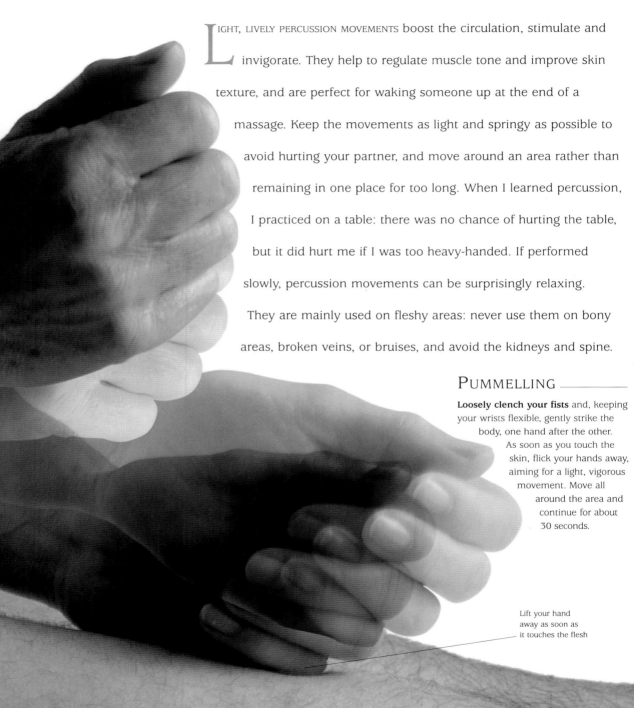

L IGHT, LIVELY PERCUSSION MOVEMENTS boost the circulation, stimulate and invigorate. They help to regulate muscle tone and improve skin texture, and are perfect for waking someone up at the end of a massage. Keep the movements as light and springy as possible to avoid hurting your partner, and move around an area rather than remaining in one place for too long. When I learned percussion, I practiced on a table: there was no chance of hurting the table, but it did hurt me if I was too heavy-handed. If performed slowly, percussion movements can be surprisingly relaxing. They are mainly used on fleshy areas: never use them on bony areas, broken veins, or bruises, and avoid the kidneys and spine.

PUMMELLING

Loosely clench your fists and, keeping your wrists flexible, gently strike the body, one hand after the other. As soon as you touch the skin, flick your hands away, aiming for a light, vigorous movement. Move all around the area and continue for about 30 seconds.

Lift your hand away as soon as it touches the flesh

HACKING

Use the sides of alternate hands
to strike the body lightly and briskly.
Concentrate on the upward movement,
flicking your hands away as soon as they
touch the skin, and keeping both hands
relaxed so that your fingers knock
together. Continue this action for
about 30 seconds, moving your
hands quickly from one spot to
the next and never remaining
in the same place for too long.

PUMMELLING & HACKING

BEST FOR *Back, hips, thighs*
LEVEL ★★   OIL ✗
EFFECT *Stimulating if fast;
relaxing if slow*

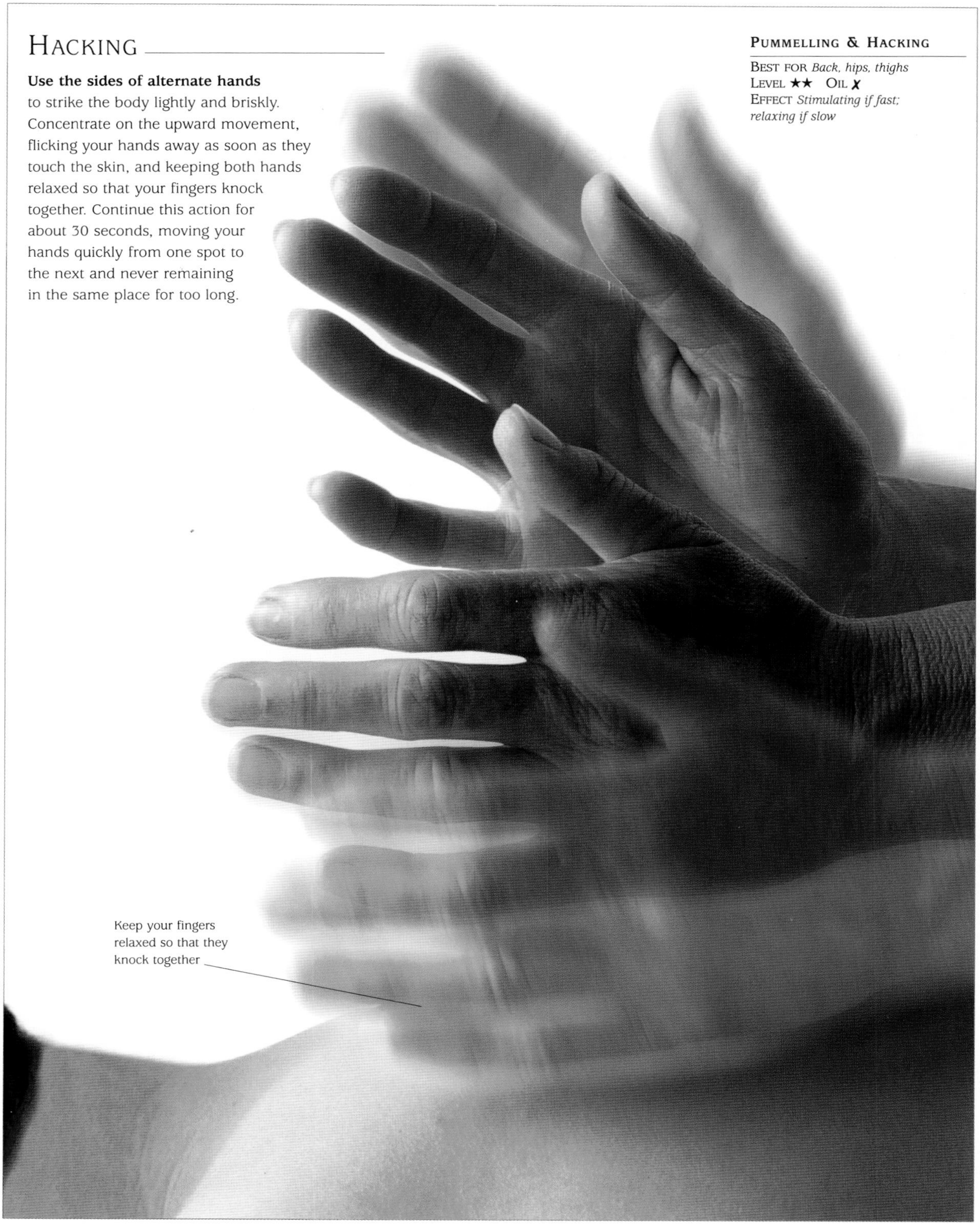

Keep your fingers
relaxed so that they
knock together

PLUCKING

Use the thumb and fingertips of alternate hands to pluck and pinch the skin briskly. This stimulates the nerve endings in the skin and can be both invigorating and surprisingly relaxing. In some traditional forms of massage, for example in Tunisia, this plucking movement is used for a complete body massage.

PLUCKING
BEST FOR *Whole body*
LEVEL ★★   OIL ✗
EFFECT *Light and invigorating*

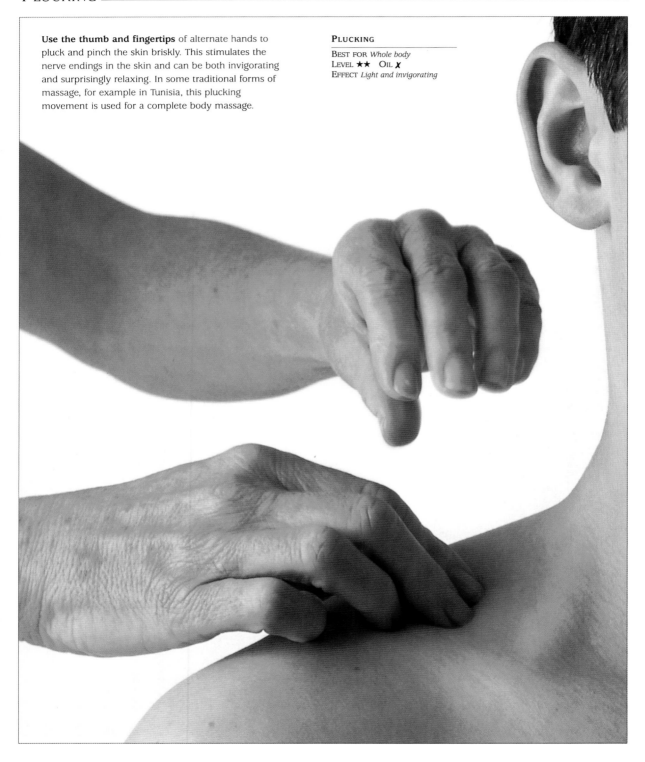

CUPPING

Cup your hands with your fingers pointing downward, and pat the area with alternate hands. This movement is softer than pummelling (*see page 40*) and can be used to relieve congested areas. Its lovely, hollow sound is particularly enjoyed by children.

CUPPING

BEST FOR *Back, buttocks*
LEVEL ★★   OIL ✗
EFFECT *Stimulating; helps relieve congested areas*

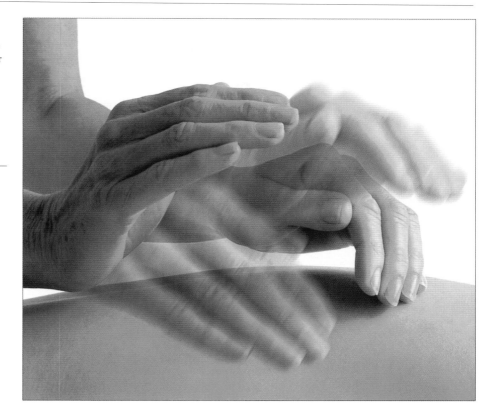

FINGER TAPPING

Rhythmically tap the fingertips of both hands on the body using an energetic, galloping motion. The movement can be superficial or deep, but it should never be heavy. Try using flat fingers to vary the effect. If working on the face, keep the movements very gentle around the eyes.

FINGER TAPPING

BEST FOR *Face, scalp*
LEVEL ★★   OIL ✗
EFFECT *Energizing*

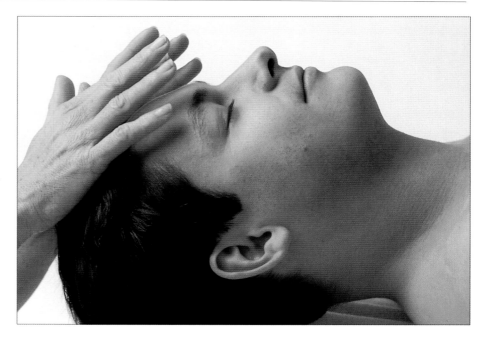

VIBRATIONS

THE FOLLOWING TECHNIQUES HELP TO RELEASE TENSION at the start or end of a massage by sending relaxing vibrations through the body. They include energetic shaking of the limbs; fine, trembling strokes along the surface of the skin; and comforting, rocking movements. Shaking and rocking are simple to master and fun to perform; superficial vibrations are difficult to learn and require perseverance, but are well worth the effort.

SHAKING

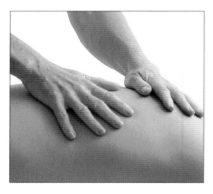

◄ **To shake an area** such as the back, stabilize the body with one hand and use your other hand to shake the flesh from side to side. You can make this movement either superficial or quite strong.

► **To shake an arm** or leg, hold the wrist or ankle firmly, taking care not to drag the skin, and shake it up and down and from side to side. Imagine you are sending waves of relaxation through the body.

SHAKING

BEST FOR *Back, legs, arms*   LEVEL ★   OIL ✗
EFFECT *Releases accumulated tension*

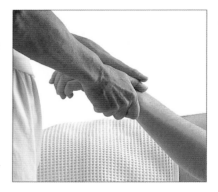

ROCKING

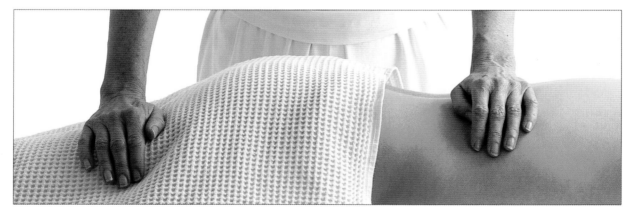

This calming movement is one of the most effective ways to relax someone. Rock the whole body by placing one hand on the back, beside the spine, and the other hand at the top of the thigh. Press into the muscles, then gently pull back and forth, building up a steady rocking motion. To rock an arm or leg, stabilize the area with one hand and rock the limb with the other hand, so that only one hand is creating the movement. Keep the rocking smooth and rhythmic.

ROCKING

BEST FOR *Whole body*
LEVEL ★   OIL ✗
EFFECT *Releases physical and emotional tension*

SUPERFICIAL VIBRATIONS

This profoundly soothing movement is only skin-deep, yet has an effect
that is felt throughout the whole body. The fine vibrations affect the nerves
and release tension just below the surface of the skin. Pull the fingers of
one hand back with the other and alternately contract and relax the
muscles of your lower forearm to create a subtle vibration.
Gradually pull your hands toward you in a gentle,
tremulous motion. Do not worry if it takes
a while to master this stroke.

ALTERNATIVE METHOD

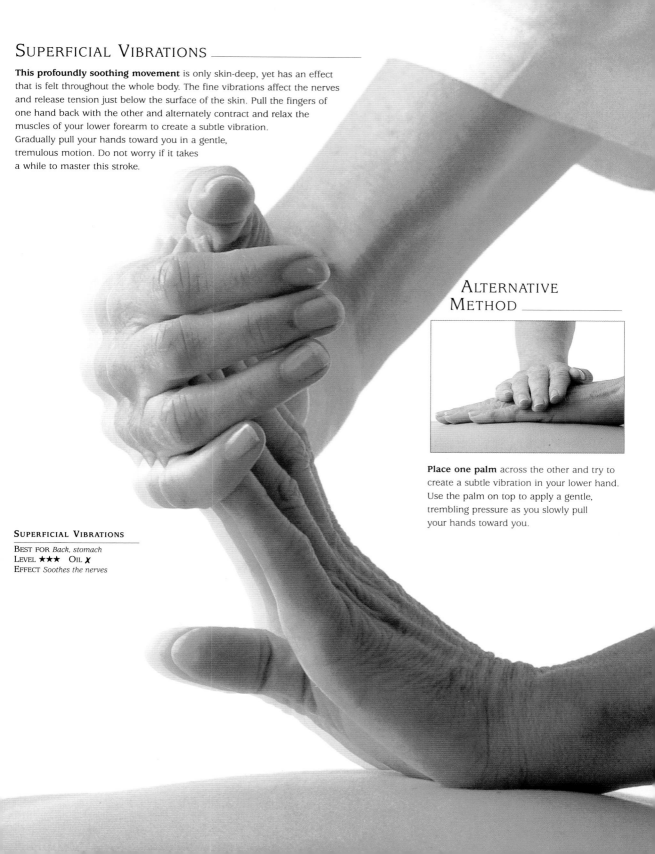

Place one palm across the other and try to
create a subtle vibration in your lower hand.
Use the palm on top to apply a gentle,
trembling pressure as you slowly pull
your hands toward you.

SUPERFICIAL VIBRATIONS

BEST FOR *Back, stomach*
LEVEL ★★★   OIL ✗
EFFECT *Soothes the nerves*

HOLDS

SIMPLE, POSITIVE HOLDS PROVIDE MOMENTS OF STILLNESS in a massage. They can be used at the start to say hello with the hands; in the middle of a massage to connect one part of the body to another; or at the end, as a farewell gesture. The aim is to communicate feelings of empathy and support. Confidence is vital, since your partner will subconsciously pick up on an unsure touch. Healing therapies such as Reiki and Polarity Therapy, which draw on Eastern medical traditions, use this kind of purposeful touch to help maintain a balanced flow of energy in the body.

INITIAL HOLDS

To accustom your partner to your touch at the start of a massage, lay your hands on the area you wish to start on and hold for about ten seconds. Relax, focusing your attention on your partner, then gradually lift your hands away.

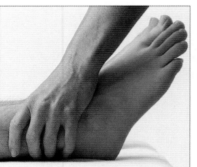

CONNECTING HOLDS

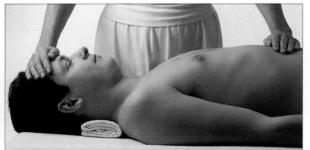

Holding each hand on a different area of the body for a few seconds during a massage can be immensely comforting for your partner. Try holding your hands on the forehead and stomach; the base of the neck and sacrum; or the hip and ankle.

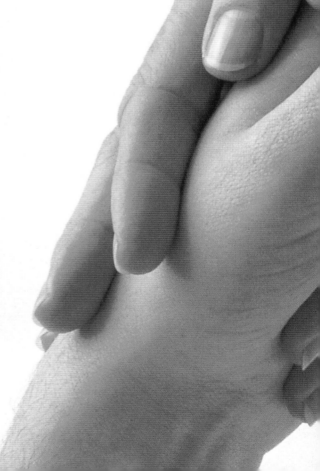

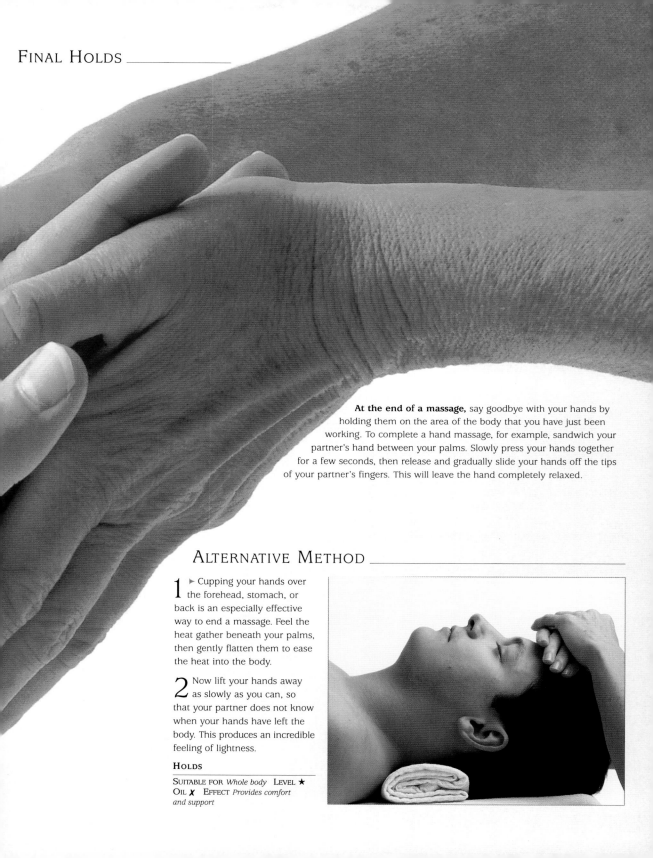

At the end of a massage, say goodbye with your hands by holding them on the area of the body that you have just been working. To complete a hand massage, for example, sandwich your partner's hand between your palms. Slowly press your hands together for a few seconds, then release and gradually slide your hands off the tips of your partner's fingers. This will leave the hand completely relaxed.

Alternative Method

1 ▶ Cupping your hands over the forehead, stomach, or back is an especially effective way to end a massage. Feel the heat gather beneath your palms, then gently flatten them to ease the heat into the body.

2 Now lift your hands away as slowly as you can, so that your partner does not know when your hands have left the body. This produces an incredible feeling of lightness.

Holds

Suitable for *Whole body* Level ★
Oil ✗ Effect *Provides comfort and support*

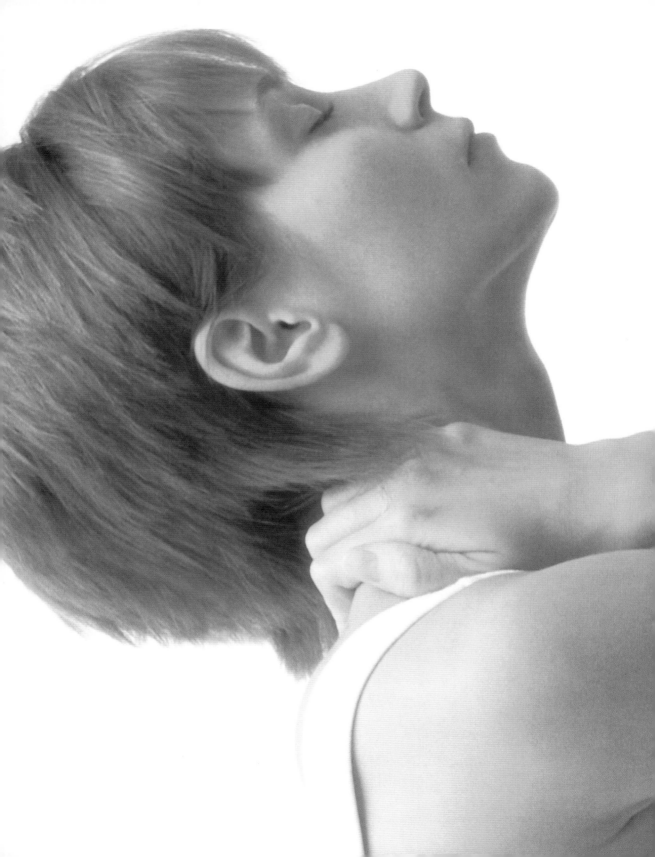

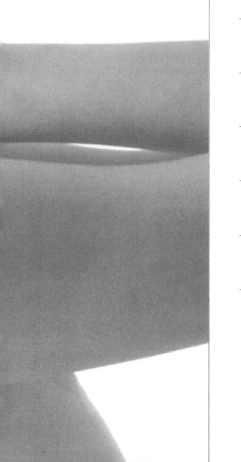

SELF-MASSAGE

MASSAGE CAN BE FOR YOURSELF AS WELL AS FOR OTHERS.

YOU CAN BE YOUR OWN LABORATORY, AND EXPERIMENT

WITH ALL THE DIFFERENT STROKES, STYLES, AND PRESSURES.

BY PRACTICING ON YOURSELF, YOU CAN DISCOVER HOW

YOUR HANDS MIGHT FEEL ON OTHERS. YOU CAN ALSO

EFFECTIVELY SOOTHE AWAY YOUR OWN TENSIONS OR PAIN,

ENERGIZE YOURSELF FOR A NEW DAY, OR PERHAPS CALM

YOURSELF WITH A MEDITATIVE MASSAGE BEFORE YOU SLEEP.

SELF-MASSAGE

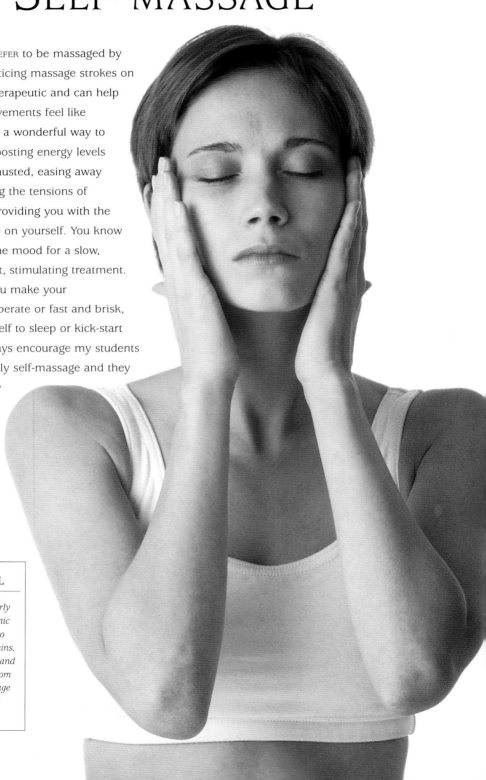

ALTHOUGH MOST OF US PREFER to be massaged by someone else, practicing massage strokes on yourself is often just as therapeutic and can help you to learn what the movements feel like to receive. Self-massage is a wonderful way to give yourself a present, boosting energy levels when you are feeling exhausted, easing away aches and pains, banishing the tensions of the day and, best of all, providing you with the opportunity to spend time on yourself. You know best whether you are in the mood for a slow, soporific massage or a fast, stimulating treatment. Depending on whether you make your movements slow and deliberate or fast and brisk, you can either send yourself to sleep or kick-start yourself into action. I always encourage my students to give themselves a weekly self-massage and they are often surprised at how good it feels. Try to choose a quiet area where you will not be disturbed, and sit in a chair or on the floor, or lie down. Then close your eyes and massage those cares away.

PAIN CONTROL

Self-massage can be particularly useful if you suffer from chronic or short-term pain. It helps to stimulate the release of endorphins, the body's natural pain-killers, and diverts your attention away from the pain. Above all, self-massage gives you a sense of control (see pages 156–157).

FACE & SCALP

The face and scalp are especially suited to self-massage: we instinctively stroke away headaches, and naturally hold our foreheads when concentrating. The scalp can store a surprising amount of tension – if it is relaxed, you should be able to move the skin fairly easily.

The face contains an enormous number of nerve receptors (*see pages 162–163*), and therefore face massage can have profound effects throughout the body, changing our moods, enhancing relaxation, and controlling pain. Remove contact lenses before you begin.

Starting at the face and working slowly down the body has a calming effect; for an invigorating self-massage, start at the feet and work upward with more energetic movements.

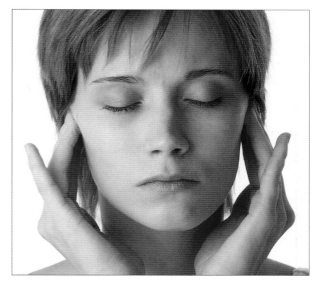

1 ◄ Stroke your whole face with soft, molding hands. Then, with the fingers of both hands, stroke slowly and firmly from the center of the forehead out to the temples. Stroke under the cheekbones, from the nose to the ears: this can help if you suffer from sinus congestion. Then stroke from the mouth to the edge of the jaw.

2 ► Explore your face with circular finger pressures, moving the skin against the underlying muscles. Vary the size, depth, and direction of the circles; try flat, shallow circles and deep, penetrating spirals. Feel for any taut, over-used muscles and pay particular attention to the jaw, as tension is frequently stored there.

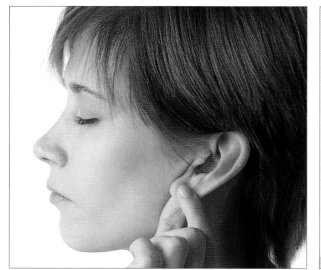

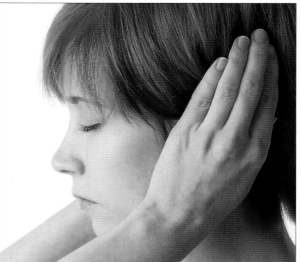

3 Gently squeeze and pull the ears with the thumb and forefinger, working around all the nooks. In traditional Chinese medicine, stimulating reflex points on the ear is said to affect the whole body.

4 Place one palm over each ear, then slowly and gently circle the ears back and down, easing pressure on the upward movement. The noise made resembles that of the sea and is very comforting.

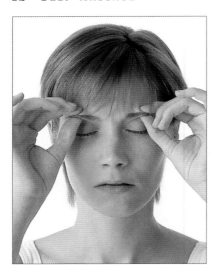

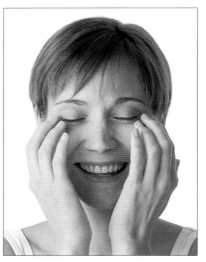

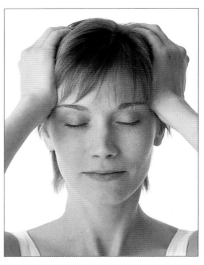

5 Gently stroke around your eyes, then squeeze along each eyebrow from the bridge of the nose to the temples with your index fingers and thumbs. If you find a sensitive spot, hold until the pain eases.

6 Use the pads of your fingers to tap under your eyes and over your eyelids. This helps to disperse congestion in the area and reduce puffiness. The feeling should resemble light rain drops.

7 Place your palms on your temples, with your fingers resting on your head, and slowly circle your palms ten times one way and ten times the other way. Then make circular palm pressures all over the scalp.

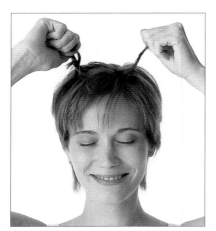

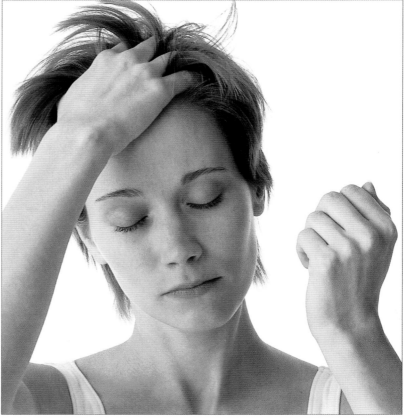

8 Clasp a handful of hair at the root in each hand, twist it around your fingers, and gently pull it. Imagine you are pulling out tension. Hold for a few seconds, then release and repeat over the scalp, using both hands together or one hand after the other.

9 Comb the fingers of one hand through the hair from the roots to the ends, then follow with the other hand. Work all over the head, trying to achieve a smooth, fluid rhythm. Take care not to hurry this movement – it can be surprisingly relaxing.

10 Use percussion movements on the head to wake yourself up. Use the fingers and thumbs of alternate hands to pluck the scalp, or pummel the area with relaxed fists. Vary the lightness and speed.

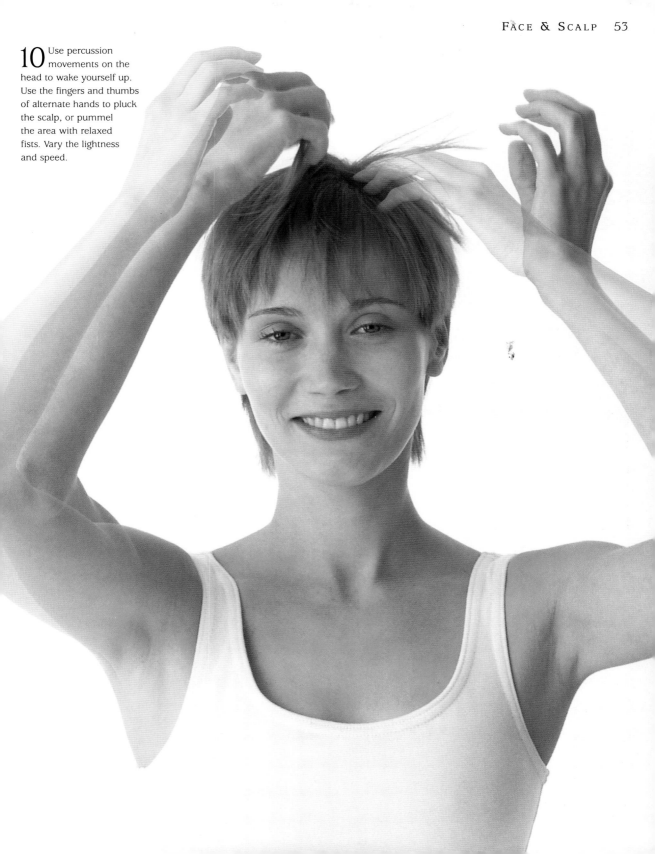

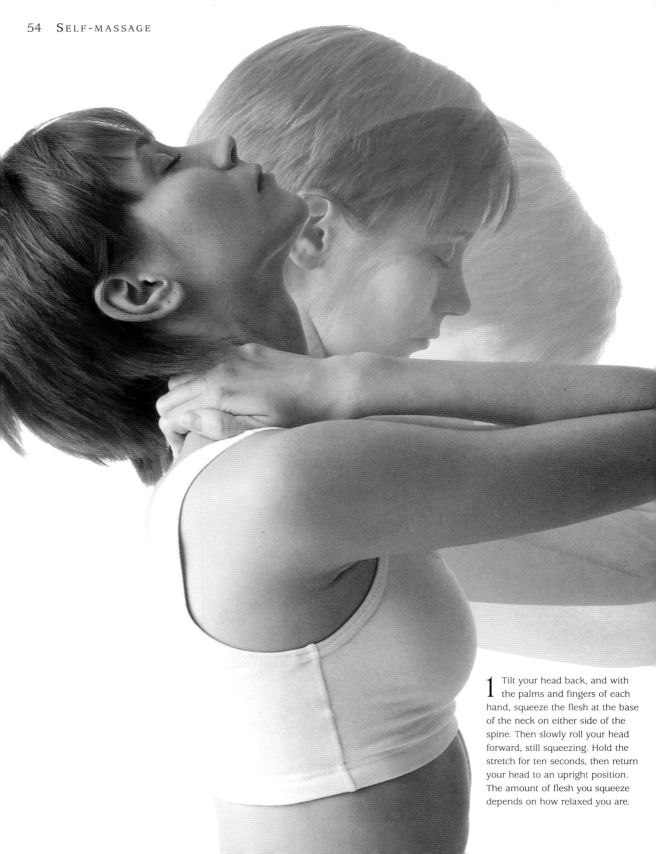

1 Tilt your head back, and with the palms and fingers of each hand, squeeze the flesh at the base of the neck on either side of the spine. Then slowly roll your head forward, still squeezing. Hold the stretch for ten seconds, then return your head to an upright position. The amount of flesh you squeeze depends on how relaxed you are.

NECK & SHOULDERS

Most people suffer tension from time to time in the neck, shoulders, and chest area, and it is useful to have a remedy literally at your fingertips! Our heads are heavy, and it is no wonder that our necks often feel strained, with the muscles becoming taut and rope-like.

Bad posture, carrying heavy bags, and slouching can exacerbate the problem. Focus on the areas that feel most tense, and work slowly and deeply. The following simple massage and exercise is an effective way of relieving tension, and can be done anywhere.

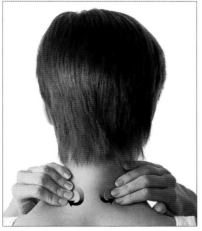

2 Stroke your hands up and down the back of the neck to warm the area. Then use the fingers of both your hands to make deep, circular pressures all around the neck area, making sure that you do not apply pressure to the spine itself.

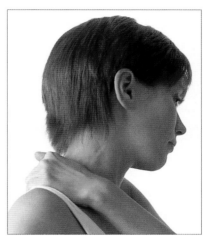

3 ▸ Place your left hand on your right shoulder and squeeze the muscle there. Hold the squeeze and slowly rotate your shoulder backward. A grinding noise indicates that the muscles are tense and should be freed up. Repeat with the right hand on the left shoulder.

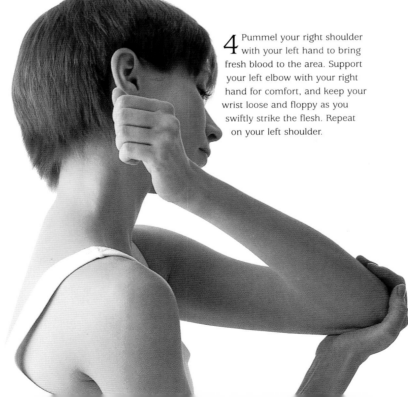

4 Pummel your right shoulder with your left hand to bring fresh blood to the area. Support your left elbow with your right hand for comfort, and keep your wrist loose and floppy as you swiftly strike the flesh. Repeat on your left shoulder.

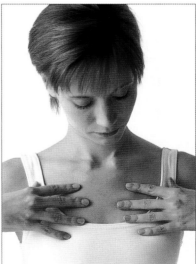

5 ▴ With your fingers, stroke firmly from the center of the chest outward, applying deep pressure between the ribs. When you reach the edges of the ribcage, return to the center and repeat. Feel for and concentrate on tense spots as you work over the chest.

LEGS & FEET

Use skin-deep strokes on the legs to encourage lymphatic drainage (*see pages 74–77*), and use deeper movements to affect the venous flow and to boost the circulation. Always stroke more firmly as you work toward the body, and use oil for fluidity. Foot massage is not only incredibly relaxing, but is believed by some practitioners, especially reflexologists, to stimulate the whole body (*see pages 98–99*).

LEGS

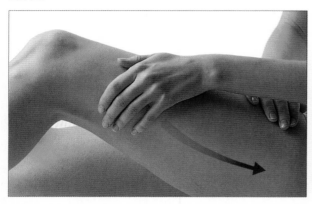

1 Start the massage by stroking your whole leg, applying a firm pressure as you stroke toward the body. You can either stroke one hand after the other, as shown here, or place one hand on either side of the leg and stroke both hands together.

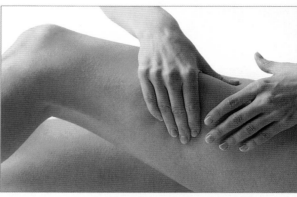

2 Now knead your leg. With alternate hands, squeeze and release the flesh at the top of your thigh, working rhythmically and thoroughly. Work all over the top of the thigh, down to the knee, and continue on the back of the thigh. Then knead the calf muscles.

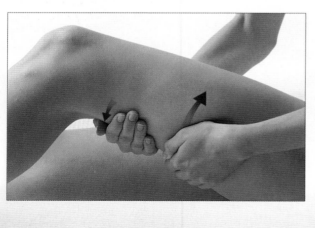

3 Soothe your leg with criss-crossing strokes. Place one hand on each side of the thigh at the knee, and pull your hands upward, squeezing the leg. Release, cross your hands over, and glide them down the other side. Then pull your hands up again to repeat. Work all the way up the thigh.

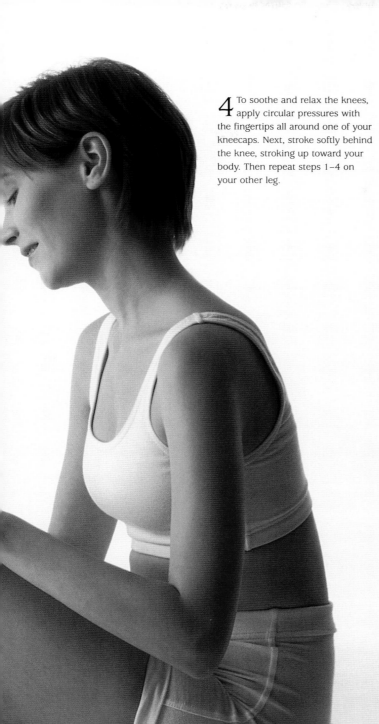

4 To soothe and relax the knees, apply circular pressures with the fingertips all around one of your kneecaps. Next, stroke softly behind the knee, stroking up toward your body. Then repeat steps 1–4 on your other leg.

FEET

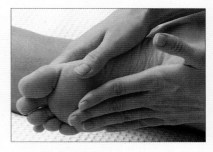

1 Rest your right foot on your left knee and sandwich the foot between your hands, fingers facing forwards. Rub your hands backward and forward along the foot to warm the whole area.

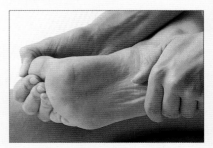

2 Support the heel of your foot with your left hand and clasp the toes with your right hand. Energetically squeeze, extend, and flex the toes to increase their flexibility.

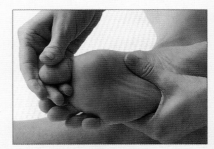

3 Still supporting the foot with your left hand, massage your toes with your right hand by squeezing, twisting, and rolling each one in turn with your fingers.

4 Place one thumb on top of the other, using your fingers to support the foot, and make deep, circular thumb pressures over the sole of the foot. Stroke the area, then repeat steps 1–4 on the left foot.

ABDOMEN & LOWER BACK

Although you can massage your abdomen while you are sitting up, it is much more relaxing, and therefore better for you, if you lie down. Lie somewhere that is comfortable, with a small pillow placed under your knees so that both your back and abdomen are relaxed.

You can massage your lower back by sitting cross-legged, as shown opposite, or by lying down on your side, with your top knee bent in front of you. The movements below are designed to release muscular tension and will aid relaxation.

ABDOMEN

1 Stroke one hand after another around your abdomen in a clockwise direction, lifting one hand over the other in a continuous flow. Increase the size of the circle to cover the whole area, then gradually make it smaller again. This clockwise stroke follows the workings of the intestine, helping to relax the abdomen, which can help to regulate digestion.

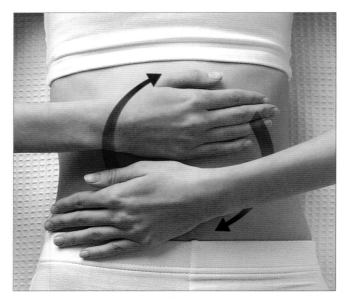

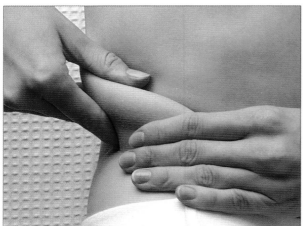

2 Bend your knees over to your left and knead the right side of your abdomen with the fingers and thumbs of alternate hands. Rhythmically pick up and release the flesh wherever you can, then bend your knees to the right and knead the left side.

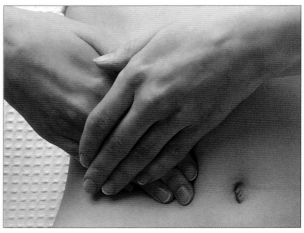

3 Apply static and circular pressures all around the abdomen, following the outline that you traced with your strokes in step 1. Use one hand on top of the other, or the palm of just one hand, according to how much pressure you want to apply.

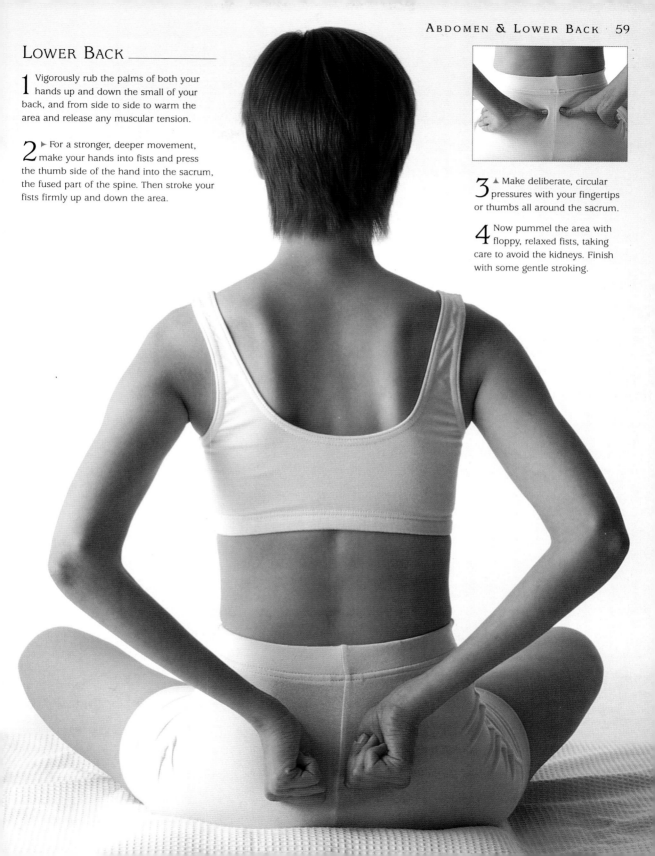

LOWER BACK

1 Vigorously rub the palms of both your hands up and down the small of your back, and from side to side to warm the area and release any muscular tension.

2 ▶ For a stronger, deeper movement, make your hands into fists and press the thumb side of the hand into the sacrum, the fused part of the spine. Then stroke your fists firmly up and down the area.

3 ▲ Make deliberate, circular pressures with your fingertips or thumbs all around the sacrum.

4 Now pummel the area with floppy, relaxed fists, taking care to avoid the kidneys. Finish with some gentle stroking.

ARMS & HANDS

Anyone who habitually uses their arms and hands, spending long periods of time at a computer, for example, or playing a racket sport, will benefit from massage in these areas. Tension in the arms can create aches and pains in the shoulders and neck, so use strong movements to unlock tightness in the upper arms and forearms. The hands contain numerous nerve endings, and massage here benefits the whole body. In reflexology (*see pages 98–99*), the hand is thought to map the body, with parts corresponding to reflex areas.

ARMS

1 Begin by stroking your whole arm from the wrist to the shoulder, working firmly as you move up the arm and then gliding gently back down again.

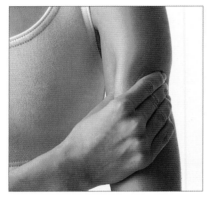

2 ▲ Now try one-handed kneading: squeeze and roll the muscles of the arm between the fingers and heel of your hand. Start kneading on the upper arm, and work down from the shoulder to the wrist.

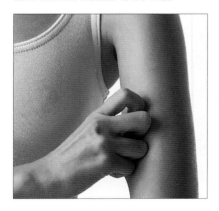

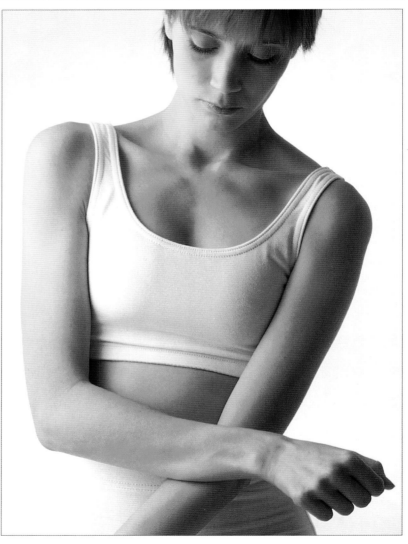

3 Use your knuckles to make rotary pressures all along the arm, working as deeply and rhythmically as you can.

4 Stroke one forearm with the other, slowly rotating the top forearm as you stroke from the elbow to the wrist of the other arm. This stroke massages both arms simultaneously, and is very effective. Repeat steps 1–4 on the other arm.

HANDS

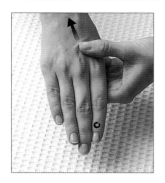

1 First, rub your palms together to warm them. Then use your thumb to stroke deeply between each tendon of one hand, from the knuckles to the wrist.

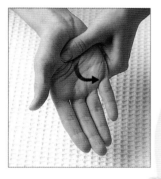

2 Stroke your thumb firmly down the palm of the hand and out to the side several times in a fanning motion. Then make deep, circular thumb pressures all over the palm.

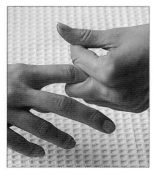

3 Pull and twist each finger in turn with the knuckles of your other hand. Work right up to the fingertips. Repeat steps 1–3 on the other hand.

FINISHING TOUCHES

Finish your self-massage with feather stroking. Start at your forehead and lightly stroke the fingertips of both hands over the face and neck, down the arms, and off at the tips of the fingers. Then stroke the front of the body, down the legs, and off at the feet. This movement should leave you feeling refreshed, calm, and as light as a feather.

> ❝ *I begin my massage feeling tired and worn down and emerge feeling like a butterfly.* ❞
> MASSAGE STUDENT

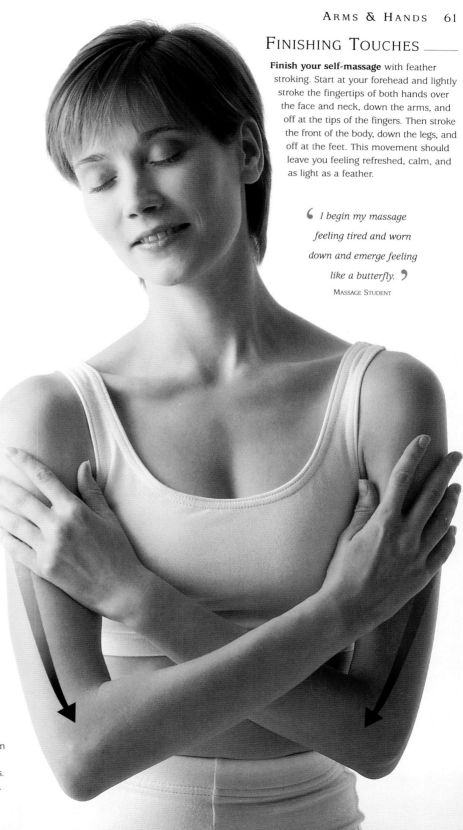

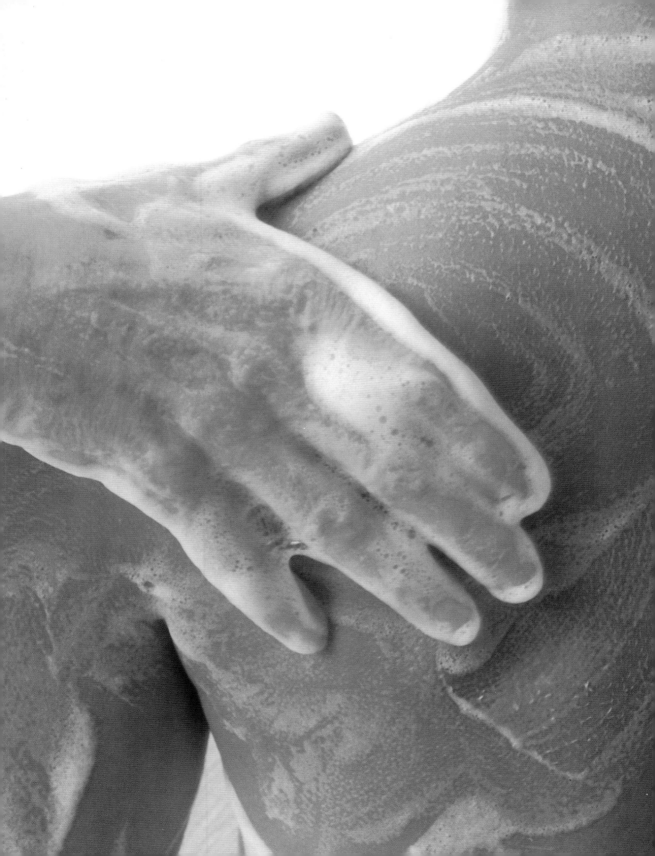

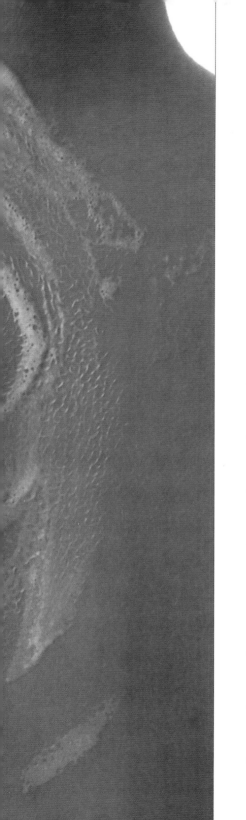

MASSAGE MASTER-CLASSES

TOUCH, THE CURRENCY OF MASSAGE, IS ONE OF THE FIVE

FUNDAMENTAL WAYS IN WHICH HUMAN BEINGS SENSE

AND EXPERIENCE THE WORLD. THROUGH TOUCH WE CAN

COMFORT, COMMUNICATE, EXPRESS LOVE, SOOTHE AWAY

PAIN, AND HEAL. THE PROPERTIES OF TOUCH ARE

PROFOUND, AND IN MASSAGE THEY ARE RAISED TO AN

ART THAT HAS MANIFESTED ITSELF ALL OVER THE

WORLD AND THROUGHOUT HISTORY.

SWEDISH MASSAGE

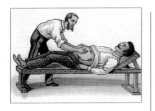

FOR A TRADITIONAL SWEDISH MASSAGE AROUND THE ABDOMEN, THE RECIPIENT'S KNEES ARE RAISED TO RELAX THE ABDOMEN MUSCLES AND THE MASSEUR WORKS IN A CLOCKWISE DIRECTION, FOLLOWING THE WORKINGS OF THE INTESTINES.

MASSAGE BECAME POPULAR in the West during the 19th century through the influence of the Swede Pir Henrik Ling (1776–1839). Ling used a knowledge of physiology to develop a system of treatment combining massage with physical exercise. This became known as Swedish Massage, and the French terms he gave some movements are still used. A sequence usually starts with *effleurage*, followed by *petrissage*, friction, vibrations, *tapotement*, *effleurage* again, and passive movements.

The aim of the Swedish treatment is, by a careful manipulation of muscles and joints, to restore to good health such as are in any way diseased.

KURRE W. OSTROM, MASSAGE AND THE ORIGINAL SWEDISH MOVEMENT, C.1885

TERMINOLOGY

EFFLEURAGE *Gliding strokes with the palms, thumbs, or fingertips.*

PETRISSAGE *Kneading movements with the hands or with the thumbs and fingers.*

FRICTION *Circular pressures with the thumbs, fingers, or palms of the hands.*

VIBRATION *Oscillatory movements that shake or vibrate the body.*

TAPOTEMENT (PERCUSSION) *Brisk pummelling, hacking, or tapping actions.*

PASSIVE & ACTIVE MOVEMENTS *Movements that are either applied to or performed by the recipient. They include bending, stretching, and rotary movements.*

KEY PRINCIPLES

Swedish massage traditionally takes place on a massage couch. Whatever surface you decide to use, it is essential that you keep your back straight throughout the massage, and that you use your body weight to achieve depth of movement. The massage usually begins on the feet and legs, followed by the hands and arms, then the abdomen and chest, and finishes on the back.

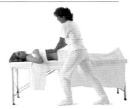

UPPER LEG

1 ▼ EFFLEURAGE With your partner lying on her back, place one hand behind the other on the thigh above the knee. Stroke both hands firmly up the front of the thigh, then glide your hands smoothly down the sides. Repeat several times.

2 PETRISSAGE Knead the thigh by lifting and then releasing the flesh with alternate hands. Work up the leg in rows so that you cover the whole area.

3 FRICTION Stabilize the leg with one hand and use the thumb or fingers of the other hand to make rows of circular pressures along the outer thigh, working from the knee up to the hip.

4 TAPOTEMENT Make a hacking movement with the sides of alternate hands along the outer thigh. Keep the action as light and brisk as possible. Then follow with *effleurage* to soothe the area.

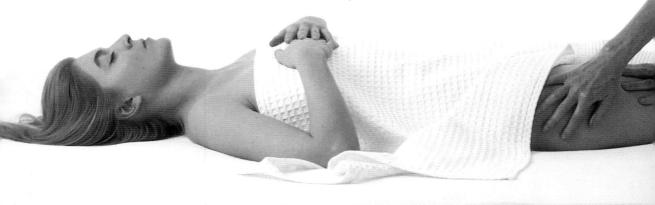

LOWER LEG

1 ▸ **FRICTION** Use one hand to support the right leg under the knee, and with the thumb of your other hand, make circular pressures all around the knee.

2 **EFFLEURAGE** Stroke firmly up the calf, from the ankle to the knee, either with one hand after the other or with both hands together.

3 **PETRISSAGE** Knead the inner calf with both hands, squeezing and releasing the flesh wherever you can. Then support the leg with one hand at the ankle, and knead the outer calf with your other hand.

4 **FRICTION** Still supporting the leg, make circular finger pressures with your other hand along the outer calf. Stroke the calf and around the ankle.

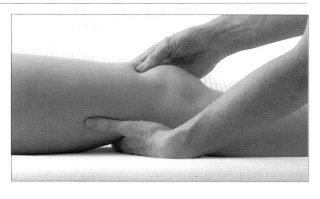

FOOT

◂ **Sandwich the foot** with your palms, then stroke firmly downward and glide back. Repeat a few times, then do some friction movements: make circular thumb pressures along the top of the foot with your fingers supporting the sole, then along the sole of the foot with your fingers holding the top. Massage each toe and finish with gentle *effleurage*.

PASSIVE MOVEMENTS

1 ▸ **FOOT ROTATIONS** Clasp the toes with one hand and support the ankle with your other hand. Slowly rotate the foot a few times, then flex the toes backward and forward.

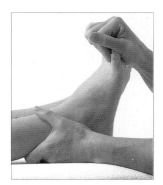

2 **LEG BENDS** Holding the ankle with one hand, raise the leg and bend the knee forward, supporting the thigh with your other hand. Straighten the leg and repeat several times. Then repeat the whole sequence for the leg and foot on your partner's other leg.

ARMS & HANDS

Follow the sequence that you used on the legs and feet, adapting the movements to accommodate the smaller surface areas of the arms and hands. Start on the upper arm, continue around the elbow and forearm, and finish with the hand. The passive movements (*see above*) can also be adapted for the arms and hands.

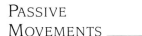

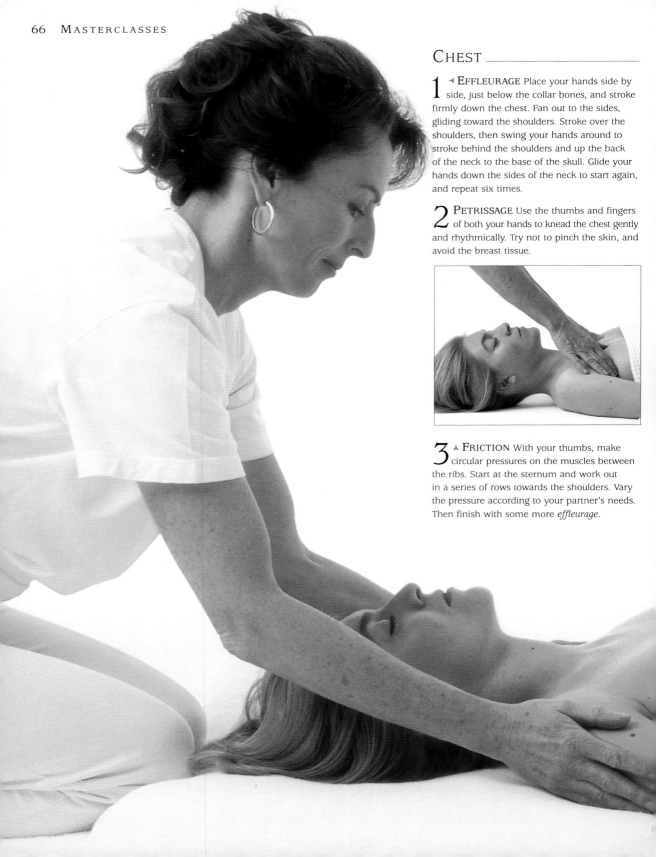

CHEST

1 ◄ EFFLEURAGE Place your hands side by side, just below the collar bones, and stroke firmly down the chest. Fan out to the sides, gliding toward the shoulders. Stroke over the shoulders, then swing your hands around to stroke behind the shoulders and up the back of the neck to the base of the skull. Glide your hands down the sides of the neck to start again, and repeat six times.

2 PETRISSAGE Use the thumbs and fingers of both your hands to knead the chest gently and rhythmically. Try not to pinch the skin, and avoid the breast tissue.

3 ▲ FRICTION With your thumbs, make circular pressures on the muscles between the ribs. Start at the sternum and work out in a series of rows towards the shoulders. Vary the pressure according to your partner's needs. Then finish with some more *effleurage*.

ABDOMEN

1 EFFLEURAGE Place a small pillow under your partner's knees to relax the abdomen. Then, facing across the body, place one of your hands on the lower ribs and the other below the navel. Stroke the lower hand slowly and lightly around the navel, working in a clockwise direction, while the other hand acts as a support. This simple movement is extremely soothing.

2 FRICTION Use the fingers of one hand to apply gentle, circular pressures, again following a clockwise direction. Support the abdomen with your other hand, and work around the navel, covering the whole of the abdominal area. Work slowly and thoughtfully. Gradually increase the pressure of your hands as your partner relaxes into the massage.

3 ▶ PETRISSAGE Knead the top of the abdomen with flat palms by rhythmically pushing whatever flesh there is in the area from hand to hand, using alternate hands. Then knead each side of the abdomen with a deeper, more stimulating movement, lifting and squeezing the flesh with one hand, and then with the other.

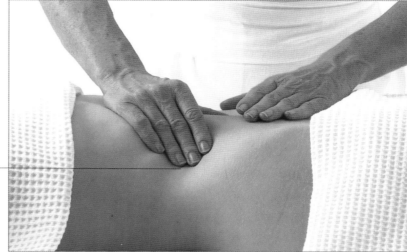

Push the flesh from one hand to the other

4 VIBRATIONS Place one palm on top of the other, below the rib cage and on the left side of the abdomen. Contract your upper forearm to create a trembling movement in your hands, then slowly pull your hands down towards the pelvis. Glide your hands across the abdomen and continue the vibrations up the right side, so that the whole movement is clockwise.

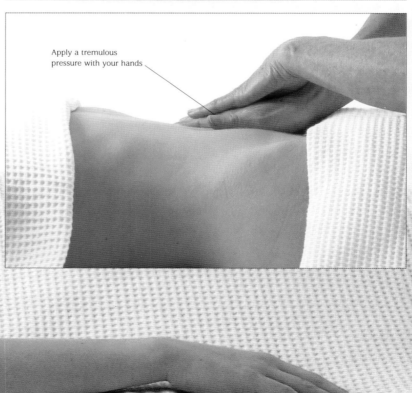

Apply a tremulous pressure with your hands

BACK

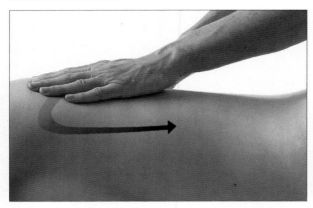

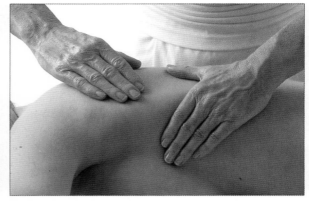

1 EFFLEURAGE Start with some gentle fan stroking. Place your hands on the lower back, on either side of the spine, and stroke firmly upward. When you reach the lower ribs, fan your hands outward, shaping your fingers around the body, and glide lightly down the sides. Repeat the movement a few times, fanning your hands out a little higher on the back each time, until you reach the shoulders. This is a lovely flowing stroke.

2 PETRISSAGE Face the body, then grasp, squeeze, and release as much flesh as you can with alternate hands. Start on the far hip, then work up the side of the back and across the shoulders, adapting your hands to suit the area. Continue on the side nearest to you: either lean down so that you can push up with your hands or move to the other side of your partner and reach across. Work twice around the back.

3 FRICTION Support the left shoulder blade with your right hand and make circular pressures with the fingers or thumb of your left hand in the groove beside the spine. Direct the pressure away from the spine. Release and repeat a little further down the back, applying a deep but relaxed pressure. Work all the way down the side of the back, carefully avoiding the spine. When you reach the hips, release, glide up, and start again on the right side of the back.

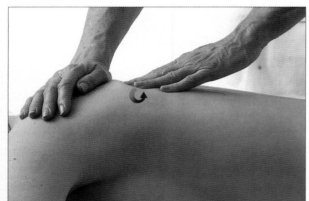

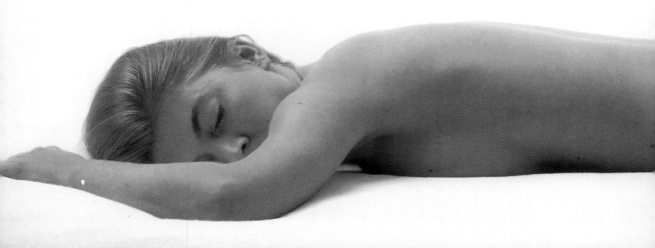

4 ▼ TAPOTEMENT Loosely cup your hands and, with the fingers pointing downward, rhythmically and lightly pat one hand after the other all over the buttocks, moving swiftly over the area. This cupping movement should make a loud, hollow sound. Continue all over the back, taking care to avoid the kidneys. You can also try hacking with the sides of your hands on either side of the spine, working up and down the back from the sacrum to the neck.

5 EFFLEURAGE Finish by stroking one hand after the other down the back. Vary the movement, depending on the effect you wish to achieve. You can either stroke lightly and quickly for a stimulating effect or slowly and soporifically to soothe and calm.

ACTIVE MOVEMENTS

In 19th-century Swedish massage, the recipient was encouraged to perform a series of systematic exercises, or active movements, in order to stimulate circulation, digestion, and respiration. Techniques included bending and stretching movements as well as "rotations" and "extensions."

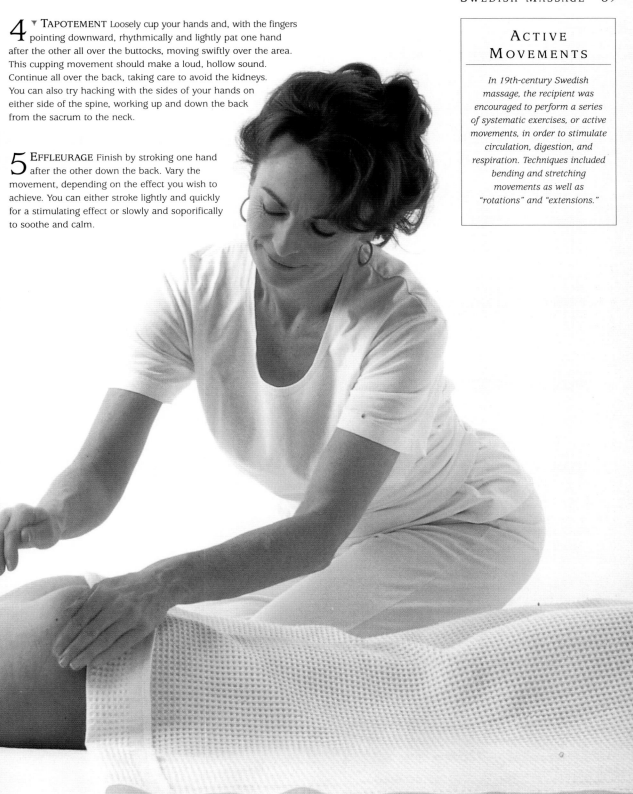

ON-SITE MASSAGE

THE ADVANTAGE OF ON-SITE MASSAGE is that it can be performed anywhere. I have massaged people in offices where the telephones are ringing incessantly, in hospital waiting rooms, and at crowded parties. Even in these busy environments, massage has worked its magic. On-site massage is particularly popular in North America, where stress-related conditions such as headaches, high blood pressure, and chronic pain account for an estimated 50 percent of absences from work a year. The techniques described below help to release the tension that can accumulate in the back and shoulders, ease aches and pains in the hands and arms after intensive computer work and, above all, help to lower stress levels. Ask your partner to loosen any tight clothing before you start. The massage takes about 15 minutes.

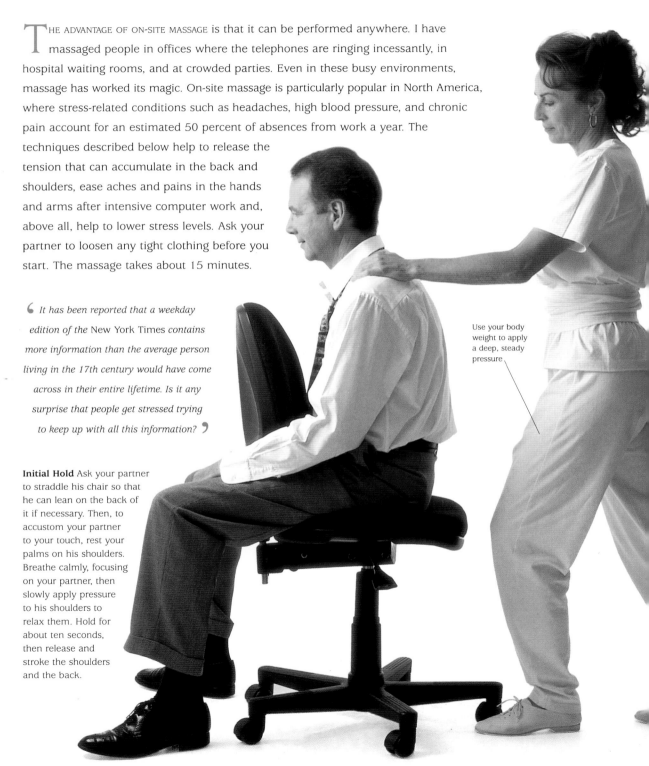

Use your body weight to apply a deep, steady pressure

It has been reported that a weekday edition of the New York Times *contains more information than the average person living in the 17th century would have come across in their entire lifetime. Is it any surprise that people get stressed trying to keep up with all this information?*

Initial Hold Ask your partner to straddle his chair so that he can lean on the back of it if necessary. Then, to accustom your partner to your touch, rest your palms on his shoulders. Breathe calmly, focusing on your partner, then slowly apply pressure to his shoulders to relax them. Hold for about ten seconds, then release and stroke the shoulders and the back.

UPPER BACK

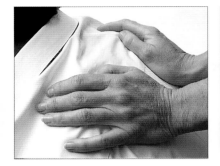

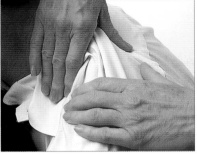

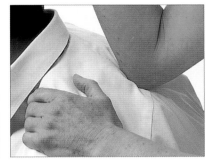

1 HEEL PRESSURES Place the heels of your hands on either side of the spine at the top of the back and apply an even pressure. Hold for a few seconds, release, and repeat at intervals down the back.

2 KNEADING Squeeze and release the muscles on the tops of the shoulders with alternate hands, pushing the flesh rhythmically from side to side. Work down the tops of the upper arms.

3 DEEP PRESSURES Support the area with your left hand and carefully apply pressure with your right elbow all around the right shoulder blade. Keep your arm relaxed so that you do not jab the flesh, then repeat on the left shoulder.

4 CIRCULAR STROKING Stroke one hand after the other in a circle around each shoulder blade in turn, to soothe the area after the elbow pressures. Lean your body weight into the heels of your hands as you stroke upward, and release the pressure on the downward movement.

5 ▶ HALF NELSON To create a deep stretch, ask your partner to place his left hand behind his back, then use your left forearm to ease his arm back. With the heel of your right hand, or your thumb, make deep pressures under the shoulder blade. Repeat on the right shoulder.

6 ◀ V-STROKES Support the forehead with one hand and with the other hand, make a "V" shape between your thumb and forefinger; stroke from the base of the neck to the skull in a scooping movement. Then, with your hands in the same position, tilt the head slowly backward and forward to stretch the muscles.

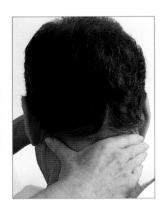

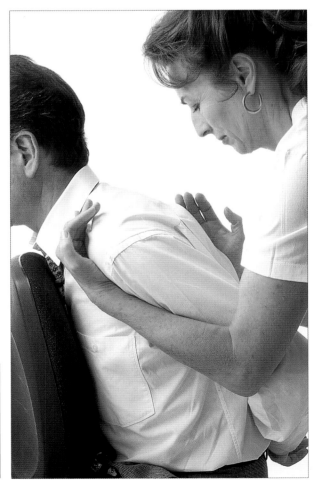

RESEARCH

Staff at the University of Miami, was either asked to relax in a reclining chair or given a 15-minute seated massage twice a week. After five weeks, the massaged staff recorded lower stress and lethargy levels, and completed mathematical problems in half the time and with half the errors of those who were not massaged.

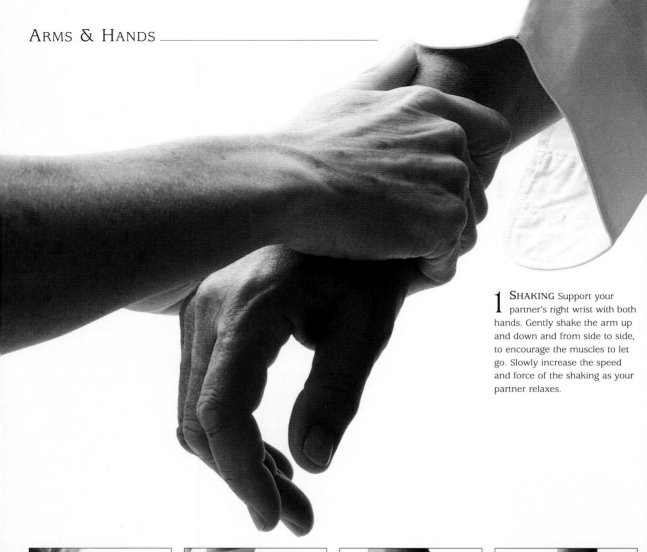

1 **SHAKING** Support your partner's right wrist with both hands. Gently shake the arm up and down and from side to side, to encourage the muscles to let go. Slowly increase the speed and force of the shaking as your partner relaxes.

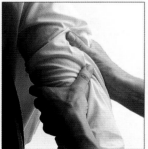

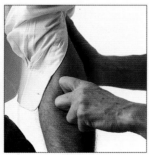

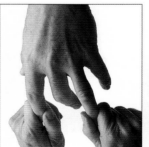

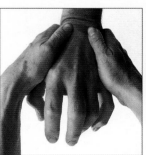

2 **KNEADING** Place one hand on either side of the right arm, near the shoulder. Squeeze and release the flesh with alternate hands, working down the arm to the wrist.

3 **KNUCKLE PRESSURES** Hold the top of the right arm with one hand and roll the knuckles of your other hand in a strong, circular motion, working up the forearm.

4 **STRETCHING THE FINGERS** Grip two fingers at the base, then squeeze and pull them, working down to the fingertips. Then repeat on the remaining fingers.

5 **FLEXING THE WRIST** Support the palm of the hand with your fingers and bend the wrist backward and forward. Then repeat steps 1–5 on the left hand.

LOWER BACK

1 CIRCULAR STROKING If your partner is wearing a belt, remove it so that you can work freely. Begin by rhythmically stroking one hand after the other in a circle around the sacrum to soothe the area.

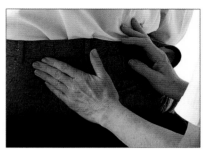

2 ▸ PRESSURES Apply deep, static and circular pressures with the fingers of one hand all around the sacrum, while the other hand supports the back. You can vary the movement by using your thumbs or the heels of your hands to apply pressure. Avoid putting pressure on the spine itself.

3 ◂ SAWING Use the sides of your hands to rub the sacrum backward and forward in a sawing motion. This is a fast, warming movement that relaxes tense muscles. Follow with gentle stroking to soothe the lower back.

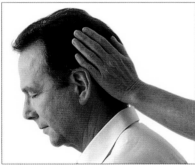

FINAL TOUCHES

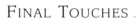

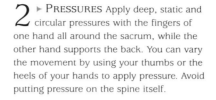

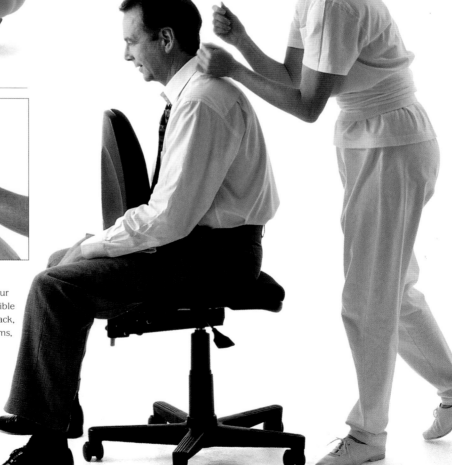

Calming down To leave your partner in a state of deep relaxation, stroke your fingertips as lightly and slowly as possible from the top of his head to the lower back, then across the shoulders, down the arms, and off at the hands.

▸ **Waking up** If your partner wishes to be left feeling ready for work, use hacking or pummelling movements to wake him up. With relaxed wrists, pound the tops of the shoulders, using alternate hands in a light, swift action.

MANUAL LYMPHATIC DRAINAGE

A GENTLE, YET POWERFUL technique that consists of slow, delicate, repetitive movements, Manual Lymphatic Drainage (MLD) was developed by Danish massage therapist Dr. Emil Vodder and his wife Estrid in the 1930s. They discovered that gently palpating and moving the skin could stimulate the lymphatic system and improve congestive conditions. This led them to develop a system to treat the whole body. The technique has many applications, from self-help treatment of minor swellings to professional treatment for chronic edema.

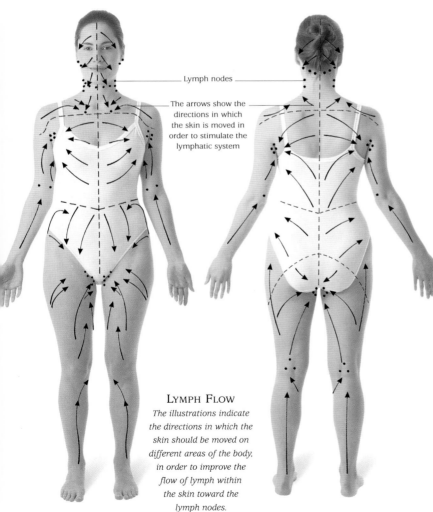

Lymph nodes

The arrows show the directions in which the skin is moved in order to stimulate the lymphatic system

LYMPH FLOW
The illustrations indicate the directions in which the skin should be moved on different areas of the body, in order to improve the flow of lymph within the skin toward the lymph nodes.

HOW MLD WORKS

The lymphatic system picks up debris and waste products from the body's connective tissue. It consists of a series of lymph nodes, connected by lymph vessels. The nodes occur in clusters, mainly around the neck, armpits, and groin; they contain white blood cells that help to fight infection by filtering out bacteria as the lymph, a watery fluid, passes through the nodes.

Healthy connective tissue nourishes every body cell, but when it is congested, cell nutrition and the flow of waste products to the bloodstream slows down. When the lymph system is stimulated by MLD, this stagnation is reversed, the body functions more healthily, and the immune system is strengthened.

WHEN TO USE MLD

MLD is a useful treatment for a variety of conditions, helping to reduce swelling and bruising, minimize scarring, and speed up healing. It can be used to relieve sinus congestion, reduce water retention and cellulite, and help ease arthritic pain. It is also a useful first-aid treatment for minor burns, knocks, and abrasions. For MLD to work successfully, it must be used frequently. Consult a qualified medical practitioner for serious or persistent conditions, such as swelling that occurs in heart failure, cancer, or recent thrombosis.

SELF-TREATMENT

Whatever condition you are treating with MLD, always begin on the neck, as this is where 30 percent of the body's lymph nodes are located. You can then work toward the area that specifically needs attention. Stationary circles are the easiest movements to use in self-treatment: the fingers remain inert, with movement coming from the arms. The sequence below is a simplified MLD treatment, designed to reduce puffiness and firm the skin. Five stationary circles are made at each point and no oil is required. The movements made should be repetitive and extremely gentle, so that the skin is only moved superficially.

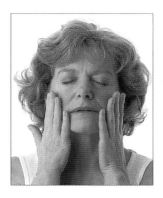

1 Raise your elbows so that they are at right angles to your body, and place your hands on either side of the neck, just below the ears. Straighten your fingers, keeping them relaxed, and use the middle part of them to circle the skin back and down as superficially as possible. Release, and let the skin gently pull your fingers upward to complete the circle. Repeat four times, then move your hands a finger-width down the neck and repeat another five times. Now cross your arms in front of your chest and make five stationary circles at the tops of the shoulders, bringing the skin forward, toward the collarbone, and releasing in toward the neck. Repeat the entire sequence three times.

2 Place your hands on either side of the jaw, and make five stationary circles at three overlapping positions, working toward the ears: move the skin down toward the body and release out towards the ears, letting the skin pull your fingers back. Repeat the sequence three times. Then make stationary circles on the rest of the face, using the length of all the fingers on the flatter areas and one or two fingers on either side of the nose.

Use just enough pressure to move the skin over the underlying tissue

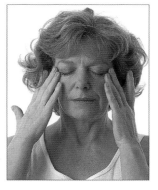

3 If you experience puffiness or discoloration under the eyes, make stationary circles in three positions along the edges of the semicircles just above the cheekbones, starting beside the nose. Use the pads of your fingers and apply half the pressure used elsewhere. Finally make stationary circles down each side of the face and repeat step 1 three more times.

TREATING A PARTNER

Because MLD is so slow and repetitive, it can have an incredibly soporific effect, and may therefore be used to calm a partner, sending them to sleep within minutes. The technique is particularly effective when used on the face. MLD takes practice to master, and the following key movements will help to direct the flow of lymph around the body. Stationary circles are used mainly on the face and painful areas; pump and scoop techniques are used on the limbs; and rotary movements are used on larger, flatter areas, such as the back and abdomen. Whichever area you focus on, always clear the neck first with stationary circles (*see page 75*).

STATIONARY CIRCLES

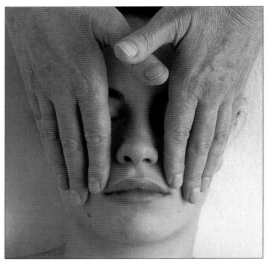

2 Place your fingers on either side of the mouth, and make five stationary circles, ensuring that your fingers are relaxed and straight. Continue with stationary circles on the rest of the face (*see page 75*).

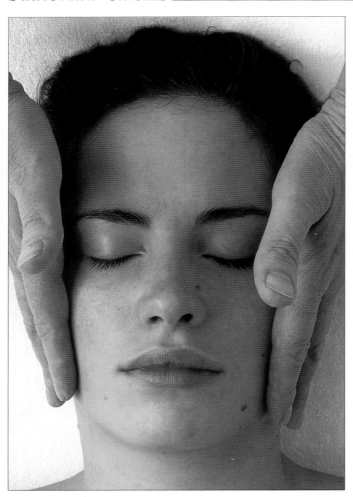

1 Place your fingers on either side of the jaw, and complete five stationary circles at three overlapping positions, working toward the ears: move the skin gently toward the body, then out to the ears, then release, allowing the skin to pull your fingers back. Repeat the sequence three times.

RESEARCH

Evidence indicates that MLD may strengthen the immune system. It is also used post-operatively to treat edemas, severe swellings in the limbs. About 25 percent of women develop edemas after breast cancer operations, and MLD, when performed by a fully qualified practitioner, can minimize the problem. Research has found that MLD reduces the swelling, improves symptoms such as pain and heaviness, and enhances the emotional well-being of the patient.

PUMP & SCOOP

1 Before working on the leg, clear the groin area with stationary circles, moving the skin toward the body. Then bend the knee and place one hand on the front of the leg and the other behind it.

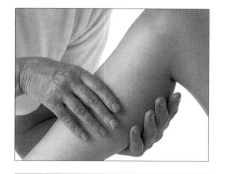

2 To perform the pump action, use your front hand to stretch the skin gently out toward each side of the leg, then ease the skin up toward the body with your palm.

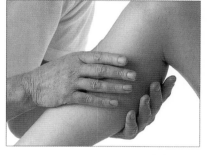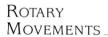

3 Follow with a scoop: use your bottom hand to push the skin upward in a light, scooping motion. Continue up to the knee with alternate pumps and scoops, doing three pumps and three scoops.

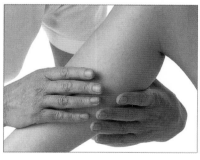

ROTARY MOVEMENTS

Place your hands on the lower back so that your thumbs are at right angles to the spine. Gently move the skin forward and out with your palms, then release and let the skin bring your hands back. Lift up your wrists, glide your fingers forward slightly, lower your palms again, and repeat. Work up the back with these rotary movements.

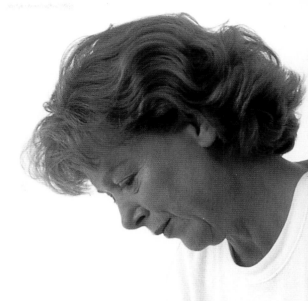

CHINESE MASSAGE

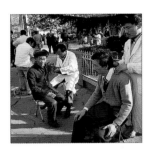

MASSAGE IS PART OF DAILY LIFE IN CHINA. HERE, BLIND MASSEURS WORK IN A STREET IN XIAN.

IN CHINA, massage is one of the centuries-old folk therapies, with acupuncture and herbal medicine, that still plays an essential part in Chinese medical care. Different systems co-exist, including *tuina* ("pushing and grasping") and *anmo* ("pressing and rubbing"), and there are numerous regional styles. In the warm south, the massage tends to be gentle and slow, while in the colder north it is strong and vigorous. Traditionally, the massage is performed through clothes.

❛ The mind of the physician and the mind of the patient should be level and in harmony, following the movements... ❜

ZHEN DA CHENG, 1601

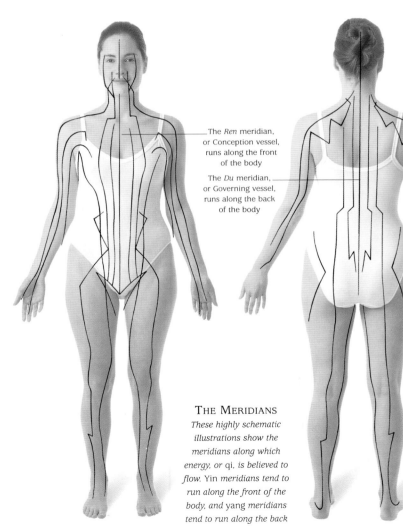

The *Ren* meridian, or Conception vessel, runs along the front of the body

The *Du* meridian, or Governing vessel, runs along the back of the body

THE MERIDIANS

These highly schematic illustrations show the meridians along which energy, or qi, is believed to flow. Yin *meridians tend to run along the front of the body, and* yang *meridians tend to run along the back*

KEY PRINCIPLES

Traditional Eastern medicine is based on the belief that life energy flows along channels, or meridians, in the body. In traditional Chinese medicine, this energy is known as *qi* and the aim of all treatments, including that of massage, is to create an unobstructed flow of *qi* in the body, thus promoting harmony and well-being. There are 12 regular meridians, each one influencing a major organ and its associated functions.

Another two meridians trace the midline of the body, *Ren* (Conception vessel) at the front and *Du* (Governing vessel) at the back.

In a healthy person, *qi* is balanced between the opposite but complementary qualities, *yin* and *yang*. *Yin* signifies darkness, cold, and passivity; *yang* signifies light, warmth, and activity. *Yin* meridians run along the front of the body, the abdomen, and the insides of the arms and legs, and *yang* meridians run mainly on the back and the outsides of the arms and legs. A massage will aim to balance the left and right sides, the top and bottom, and the front and back into a cohesive, energetic whole.

LEARNING THE TECHNIQUES

Traditionally, a Chinese masseur practices massage techniques on a bag of rice before using them on a person. This helps him to master each movement and also strengthens his hands, the idea being to reduce the bag of rice into one of flour. Here, the powerful technique of *gung fa* is demonstrated (*see also below*).

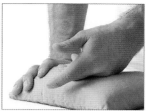

1 Place the lower knuckles of your ring and little fingers on the bag of rice.

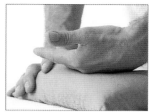

2 Roll your wrist briskly away from you in a slightly oblique direction.

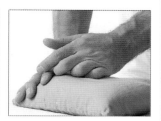

3 Now roll your wrist toward you and back on to the knuckles. Repeat until you are able to maintain a fast, strong action.

BACK MASSAGE

Although the following sequence can be performed through clothes, you may find some techniques easier if you work directly on the flesh. Adapt each step as necessary.

1 STROKING Place one hand on the sacrum, to center your partner. Stroke your other hand in a swift, smooth action up the right side of the back and around the shoulder. Glide back, then stroke up the left side of the back and shoulder in the same way.

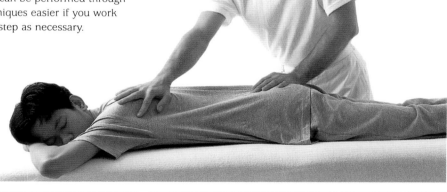

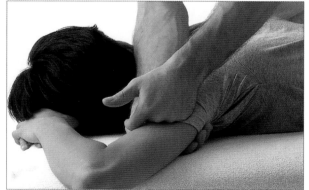

2 GUNG FA Hold the top of the arm with one hand and place the knuckles of the ring and little fingers of your other hand on top of the arm. Roll your wrist obliquely away from you, then roll it back on to the knuckles. This is a fast and powerful movement that takes a lot of practice (*see sequence, above*). Work all over the upper arm and shoulder, then repeat on the other side.

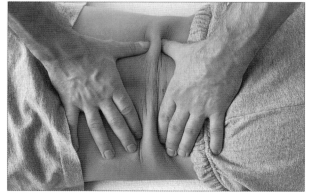

3 LUMBAR ROCKING & SQUEEZING Place your thumbs and fingertips around the muscles that run down either side of the spine at the small of the back. Then, keeping your hands still, slowly rock the body. Rock for about 30 seconds, then squeeze the flesh between your fingers and thumbs, and push your hands together to create a compression. Hold for about five seconds, then release.

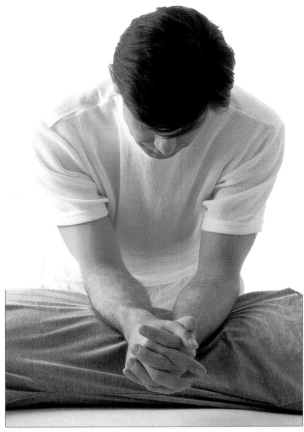

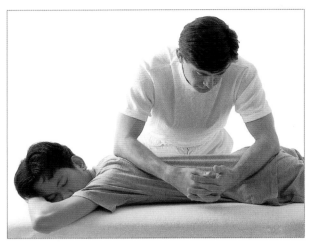

4 FOREARM KNEADING Loosely clasp your hands and rest your forearms on the upper and lower back. Then circle your forearms in an anticlockwise direction, using your body weight to achieve a deep pressure. Work slowly and systematically to cover the whole area. This technique has a warming, stretching action.

5 CHICKEN WINGING With your forearms in the same position, roll one of them briskly up and down the back while keeping the other arm still. Make sure that your body weight is evenly distributed by keeping your feet apart. Then use your other forearm to roll up the back.

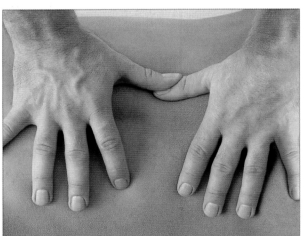

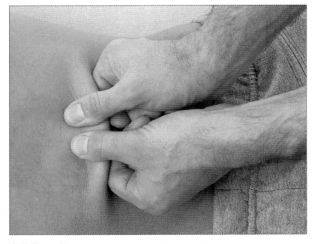

6 CROSS-FIBER WORK Place your thumbs on top of each other, just beside the spine on the side of the back nearest to you. Press down and stroke your thumbs toward the spine, with one thumb reinforcing the other. This technique will require some practice, and has a strong and tonifying effect on the muscles; stroking away from the spine relaxes taut muscles. This movement can also be done on the legs and even on the feet.

7 SKIN ROLLING Squeeze the flesh on the sacrum between your thumbs and the sides of your index fingers, and roll the flesh up the back by walking your thumbs forward. When you reach the middle of the back, glide back and repeat this movement three times. Then squeeze the flesh on the sacrum again, but instead of rolling it, pull it up sharply. This may cause a "popping" sound. Release and repeat up the back.

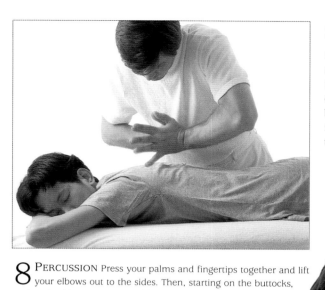

8 PERCUSSION Press your palms and fingertips together and lift your elbows out to the sides. Then, starting on the buttocks, make a hacking movement with your hands, trying to create a loud clacking sound as your fingers knock together. Work up the back, making sure that you avoid the spine.

9 SAWING In traditional Chinese massage, this vigorous movement is used in conjunction with a special warming ointment or oil. Place one hand on top of the back as a support, and make a strong, quick sawing movement with the side of your other hand, up and down the side of the spine. Repeat on the other side of the spine.

SEATED MASSAGE

For extra deep movements around the arms and shoulder area, ask your partner to sit upright, either on a couch or on a stool. You can support his back by placing your knee behind it. This is a comfortable position for both the giver and the receiver.

1 ▲ DEEP SQUEEZES Firmly grip the base of the skull on either side of the spine. With your other hand, squeeze down the arm to the wrist. Repeat about three times, then swap hands and repeat on the other arm.

2 ▲ GUNG FA This strong movement (*see page 79*) is particularly effective in this seated position. Support your partner's arm along its length with one hand and use the other hand to practise *gung fa* around the top of the arm and shoulder. Repeat on the other arm.

INDIAN MASSAGE

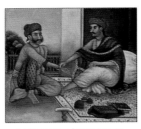

A 19TH CENTURY INDIAN PAINTING, DEPICTING AN EXAMINATION BY AN AYURVEDIC PHYSICIAN.

IN INDIA, massage is a part of everday life. If you go to the villages, you will find that almost everyone knows how to give a massage: mothers massage their babies and young children are encouraged to exchange massage with their parents and grandparents. A typical sequence may incorporate a mixture of slow, gentle strokes, brisk, invigorating movements, and warming techniques such as rubbing and squeezing.

> As food is a necessity for the organism from birth to death, so is massage to the human organism. Food provides nourishment from external sources, whereas massage excites the internal resources.
>
> HARISH JOHARI, 1984

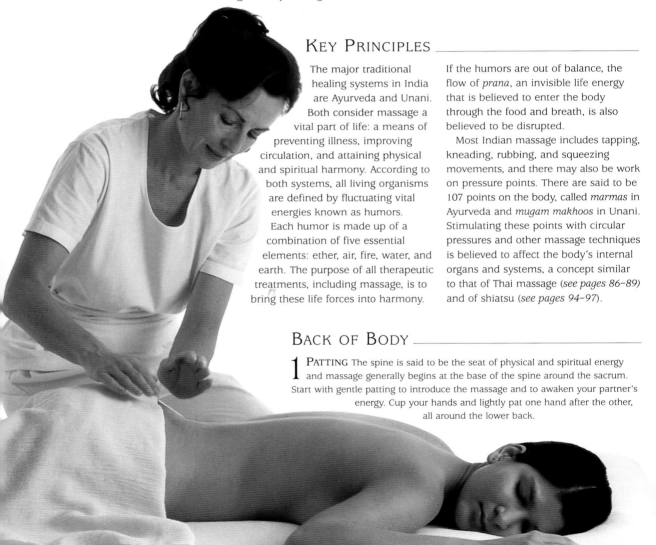

KEY PRINCIPLES

The major traditional healing systems in India are Ayurveda and Unani. Both consider massage a vital part of life: a means of preventing illness, improving circulation, and attaining physical and spiritual harmony. According to both systems, all living organisms are defined by fluctuating vital energies known as humors. Each humor is made up of a combination of five essential elements: ether, air, fire, water, and earth. The purpose of all therapeutic treatments, including massage, is to bring these life forces into harmony.

If the humors are out of balance, the flow of *prana*, an invisible life energy that is believed to enter the body through the food and breath, is also believed to be disrupted.

Most Indian massage includes tapping, kneading, rubbing, and squeezing movements, and there may also be work on pressure points. There are said to be 107 points on the body, called *marmas* in Ayurveda and *mugam makhoos* in Unani. Stimulating these points with circular pressures and other massage techniques is believed to affect the body's internal organs and systems, a concept similar to that of Thai massage (*see pages 86–89*) and of shiatsu (*see pages 94–97*).

BACK OF BODY

1 PATTING The spine is said to be the seat of physical and spiritual energy and massage generally begins at the base of the spine around the sacrum. Start with gentle patting to introduce the massage and to awaken your partner's energy. Cup your hands and lightly pat one hand after the other, all around the lower back.

2 ► GENTLE CIRCLING Use the middle fingers of one hand to make gentle circles around the sacrum. Then start to circle around the upper back between the shoulder blades with the middle fingers of your other hand. Continue for a while, keeping the movements smooth and light, then stroke the whole back.

3 THUMB PRESSURES Make deep, penetrating circles with your thumbs on either side of the spine. Start at the lower back and work up to the base of the neck in a spiraling motion.

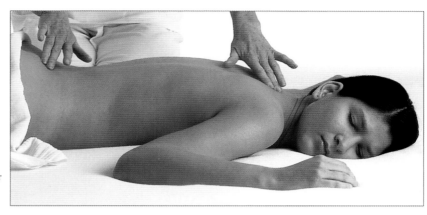

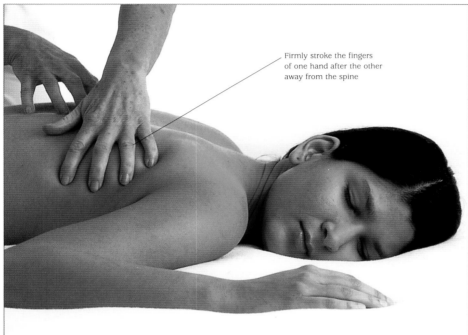

Firmly stroke the fingers of one hand after the other away from the spine

4 ◄ FINGER STROKES Begin by stroking one hand after the other strongly and slowly up one side of the back, then up the other side. Then, facing across the upper back, stroke alternate hands down the far side of the body away from the spine, spreading your fingers so that you can work deeply between the ribs. Work down to the hips, then stroke the whole area.

5 ► THUMB STROKES Now work from the shoulder and down the arm. Either kneel astride the body or lean across it from the other side. Place your fingers under the top of the arm, then push them slowly and smoothly down the arm, applying a firm pressure with your thumbs. Stroke down the whole arm and slide off at the hands. (This technique differs from Western massage, in which the strokes tend to be directed up the limbs toward the heart.) Then repeat steps 4–5 on the other side of the body.

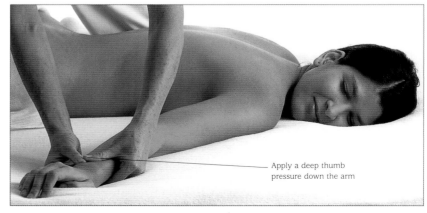

Apply a deep thumb pressure down the arm

FRONT OF BODY

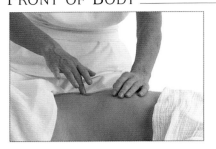

1 CIRCLING THE NAVEL Ask your partner to lie on her back with her knees bent. Place one hand on the abdomen just below the ribs. With the middle finger of your other hand stroke smoothly around the navel. In Indian massage the navel is said to be an important center of energy.

2 SIDE STROKING Use alternate hands to stroke smoothly and firmly up the far side of the abdomen. As one hand reaches the top of the area, lift it off and return it to the starting position, aiming for a rhythmic stroke. Then repeat on the other side.

3 ▶ DEEP PALM STROKES I learned this stroke from a local midwife in India. Place one hand on top of the other at hip level and stroke very slowly up the abdomen. Use your palms to maintain a deep, steady pressure and ask your partner to tell you if it is too strong. As you reach the navel, release the pressure and glide back. Repeat three times.

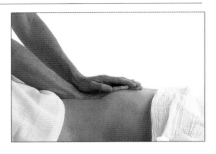

4 SOOTHING STROKES Stroke gently from the navel to the chest with both hands, then out over the ribs and down the arms. Then work on each arm in turn: use both hands to squeeze and twist the arm, working down to the fingers.

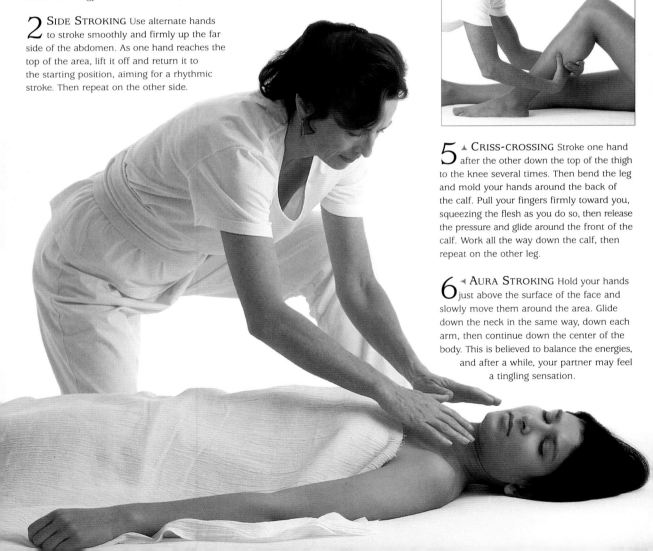

5 ◀ CRISS-CROSSING Stroke one hand after the other down the top of the thigh to the knee several times. Then bend the leg and mold your hands around the back of the calf. Pull your fingers firmly toward you, squeezing the flesh as you do so, then release the pressure and glide around the front of the calf. Work all the way down the calf, then repeat on the other leg.

6 ◀ AURA STROKING Hold your hands just above the surface of the face and slowly move them around the area. Glide down the neck in the same way, down each arm, then continue down the center of the body. This is believed to balance the energies, and after a while, your partner may feel a tingling sensation.

INDIAN BRIDAL MASSAGE

Traditionally in India, a bride and groom receive regular massage for ten days before their wedding. This is thought to aid relaxation in the bride and give a healthy glow to the skin, and to increase vigor and virility in the groom. The bride is massaged with *ubtan*, a blend of herbs, spices, and jasmine essential oil (*see recipe, below*). This leaves the skin smooth, radiant, and impregnated with the scent of jasmine.

GLOWING SKIN

Apply the *ubtan* blend all over the body with stroking and kneading movements as if you were applying a scrub. When it begins to dry, continue to rub until you remove all the paste. This will leave the skin smooth, silky, and glowing with health. After removing the paste, use plain water or rose water to wipe the skin.

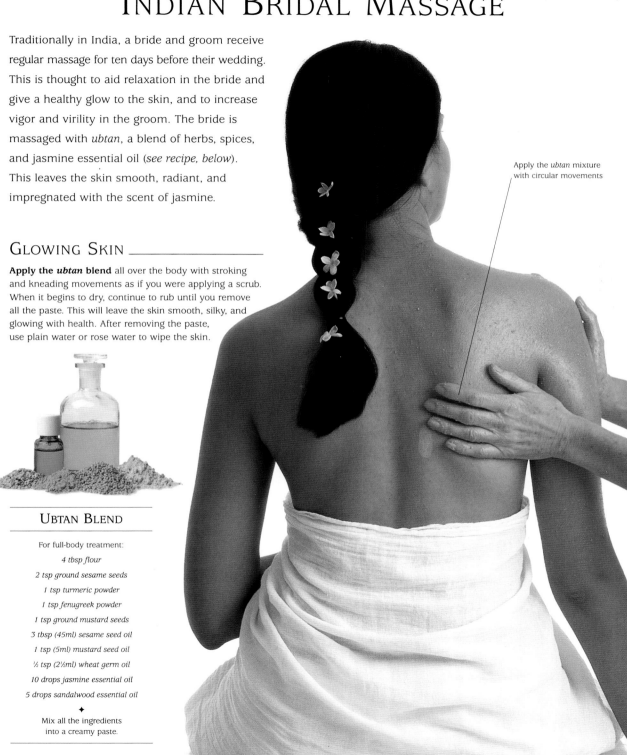

Apply the *ubtan* mixture with circular movements

UBTAN BLEND

For full-body treatment:

4 tbsp flour

2 tsp ground sesame seeds

1 tsp turmeric powder

1 tsp fenugreek powder

1 tsp ground mustard seeds

3 tbsp (45ml) sesame seed oil

1 tsp (5ml) mustard seed oil

½ tsp (2½ml) wheat germ oil

10 drops jasmine essential oil

5 drops sandalwood essential oil

◆

Mix all the ingredients
into a creamy paste.

THAI MASSAGE

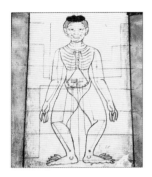

MURALS IN THE WALLS OF THE WAT PHO
TEMPLE IN BANGKOK DEPICT THE SEN
LINES USED IN THAI MASSAGE.

TRADITIONAL THAI MASSAGE is believed to have its origins in Indian medicine, with techniques handed down from teacher to pupil since the 3rd century BC. Chinese settlers may also have been influential in its development. Like other Eastern medical traditions, Thai massage is based on the concept of energy lines in the body, and it is closely connected with Buddhist teaching. It is sometimes known as Thai yoga massage because many of the stretches involved resemble yoga postures. Here, I demonstrate a few of the many movements.

> *Giving massage was understood to be a physical application of* metta, *the Pali (and Thai) word used in Theravada Buddhism to denote "loving kindness".*
>
> ASOKANANDA, THE ART OF
> TRADITIONAL THAI MASSAGE, 1996

KEY PRINCIPLES

Good health is said to depend on a balanced flow of life energy, called *prana*, through an invisible network of channels in the body. These channels are called *sen* lines and can be likened to the Chinese concept of meridians in the body (*see page 78*). Out of 72,000 *sen* lines in the body, there are ten that are considered to be the most important in Thai massage.

A Thai masseur tries to achieve perfect energy balancing by stretching the *sen* lines, and by using the hands, feet, and elbows to apply pressure to key points along them. The belief is that the physical body is the vehicle through which the emotional or psychic body can be reached. The masseur traditionally performs the massage in a meditative mood, beginning with a prayer and working with full awareness and "mindfulness". A sequence usually takes between 2 and 2½ hours.

FRONT OF BODY

This sequence begins on the legs, where there are six *sen* lines. Palm and thumb pressures are used in conjunction with stretching techniques.

1 OUTER THIGH Bend the left knee over the right thigh and hold it down with your left hand. This creates a stretch in the back. Then use your right palm to apply a series of static pressures under the thigh muscle, working up to the hips. Repeat on the right leg.

2 INNER THIGH Now place the left thigh out to the side at right angles to the body. Hold the left heel with your right hand and pull back with your body. Then, using your right foot to stabilize the thigh, "walk" the instep of your left foot along the inner thigh. Repeat on the right leg.

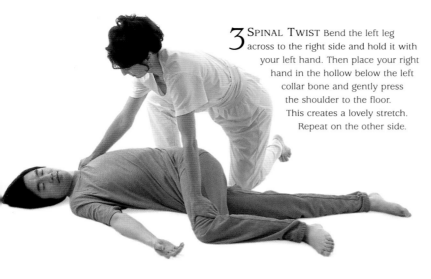

3 SPINAL TWIST Bend the left leg across to the right side and hold it with your left hand. Then place your right hand in the hollow below the left collar bone and gently press the shoulder to the floor. This creates a lovely stretch. Repeat on the other side.

PRACTICE TIPS

Before you start to massage, take time to relax and focus on your partner. Breathe slowly and deeply throughout the massage.

✦

The concept of energy channels in the body can be difficult to comprehend, especially given the different interpretations of these channels that exist between Eastern cultures. I find it helpful to imagine invisible rivers of energy that ebb and flow through the body; in some people they may be weak, in others strong. Try to use your intuition and follow their flow.

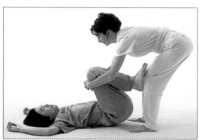

FIRST STAGE

4 STIMULATING THE KIDNEYS Stand with your feet apart and place the insteps of your partner's feet on your knees. Clasp your hands around the knees and slowly pull them toward you (*first stage*). Then move backward and downward, lifting your partner's body as you do so and keeping your back relaxed (*second stage*). Pull your partner into a shoulder stand as you move into a squatting position (*third stage*). This helps to stretch your partner's kidney lines, and stimulates kidney points on the feet.

CAUTION *Take care during this exercise: make sure that you maintain a firm grip throughout.*

SECOND STAGE

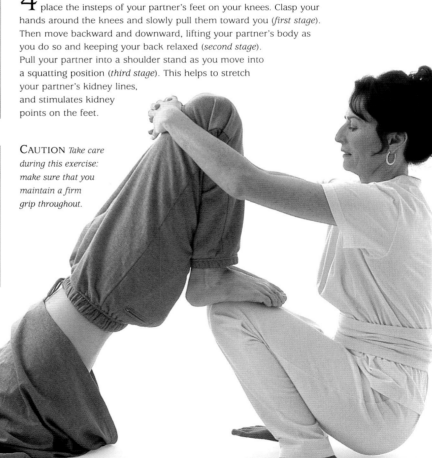

THIRD STAGE

BACK OF BODY

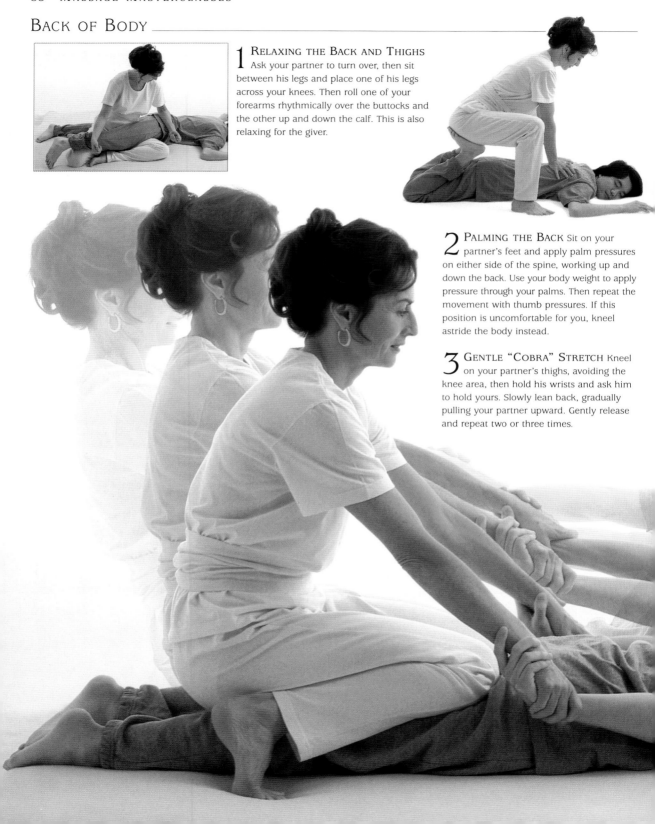

1 RELAXING THE BACK AND THIGHS
Ask your partner to turn over, then sit between his legs and place one of his legs across your knees. Then roll one of your forearms rhythmically over the buttocks and the other up and down the calf. This is also relaxing for the giver.

2 PALMING THE BACK Sit on your partner's feet and apply palm pressures on either side of the spine, working up and down the back. Use your body weight to apply pressure through your palms. Then repeat the movement with thumb pressures. If this position is uncomfortable for you, kneel astride the body instead.

3 GENTLE "COBRA" STRETCH Kneel on your partner's thighs, avoiding the knee area, then hold his wrists and ask him to hold yours. Slowly lean back, gradually pulling your partner upward. Gently release and repeat two or three times.

SEATED MASSAGE

1 COUNTER-COBRA Ask your partner to lie on his back again. Then, standing with your feet next to his buttocks, cross his legs and rest them against your shins. Grasp your partner's wrists and pull him toward you. Repeat two or three times, then slowly walk backward, pulling your partner into a sitting position.

3 LOOSENING THE SHOULDERS Stand behind your partner with your legs straight, and place your thumbs on the tops of his shoulders, near the neck. Gradually lean your body weight on to your thumbs for a few seconds, then slowly release and repeat further along the shoulders, avoiding the bony areas.

2 ARMS With your partner still in a sitting position, kneel behind him and gently pull his left elbow back with your right hand, keeping his body straight and pulling only as far as the elbow will comfortably go. Then use your left hand to squeeze up and down the arm; this squeezing stimulates the energy line along the inner arm. This area may be quite tender. Repeat on the other arm.

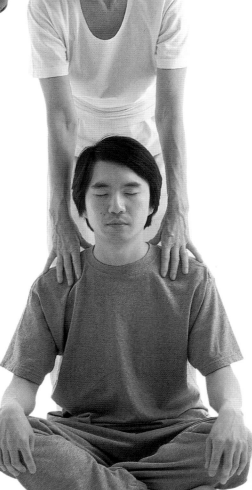

EASTERN HEAD MASSAGE

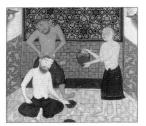

THIS ILLUSTRATION FROM A 15TH-CENTURY MANUSCRIPT DEPICTS A PERSIAN BARBER GIVING A STIMULATING HEAD MASSAGE.

HEAD MASSAGE is extremely popular throughout the East. In India, China, Singapore, and Turkey most barbers and hairdressers will automatically offer a scalp massage. In fact, the word "shampoo" derives from the Hindi word *capna,* meaning to "press" or "rub". This ten-minute massage is quite energetic and is done on dry rather than wet hair, to avoid stretching the hair. Walk around your seated partner as you work.

❛ I was taught this invigorating head massage in India. Think of the scalp as a continuation of the face, to be stroked, pressed and pampered. It will leave your partner feeling refreshed and revitalized. ❜

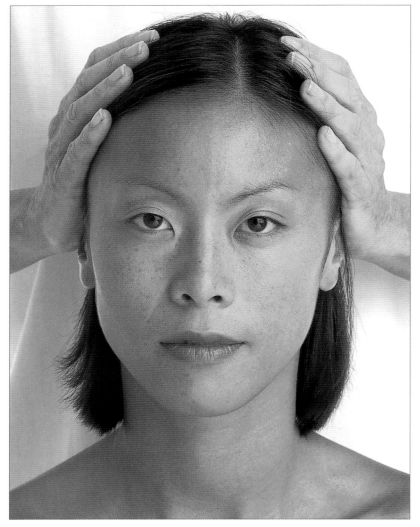

1 ◄ COMPRESSIONS To bring awareness to the area, rest your hands lightly on either side of the head with the fingers pointing upward. After about a minute, slowly press your hands toward each other, adding a very slight lift. Gradually release the pressure and repeat a few times. This simple movement is unbelievably relaxing.

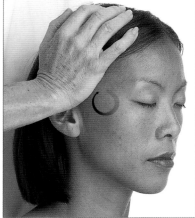

2 ▲ PALM PRESSURES Support the head with your left hand and use the palm of your right hand to apply circular pressures all over the scalp. Press into the scalp so that skin tissue, not hair, is moved. This movement feels good around the temples. Repeat the movement with your left hand, then use the palms of both hands together to lift and rotate the scalp, applying circular pressures to the sides of the head.

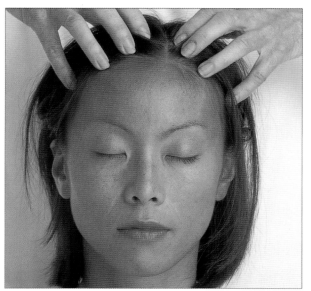

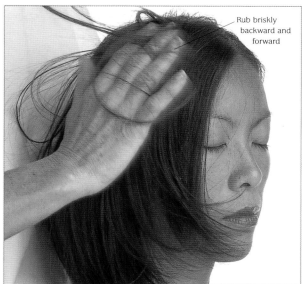

Rub briskly
backward and
forward

3 FINGER PRESSURES With relaxed, curled fingers, make circular pressures all over the scalp, from the forehead to the nape of the neck. Keep your fingers firmly in place so that you move the skin against the bone. The amount that your hands move will depend on the tightness of the scalp. Then apply static finger pressures around the base of the skull (*see pages 38–39*).

4 BRISK RUBS Support the head with your left hand again and use the flat fingers of your right hand to rub lightly and swiftly backward and forward over the head, starting behind the right ear. Work up and across, so that you cover the whole of the head. Then repeat the movement with the fingers of your left hand, using your right hand to stabilize the head.

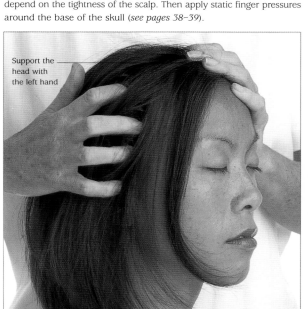

Support the
head with
the left hand

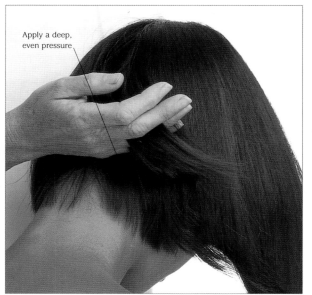

Apply a deep,
even pressure

5 ZIG-ZAGGING With the fingertips of your right hand, make short, zig-zagging movements over the scalp while your left hand supports the head. Begin by working slowly and lightly, then build up a faster, deeper action. This creates a lively, refreshing sensation. To make it more stimulating, try the same movement using your finger nails. Your partner will either love it or hate it!

6 SAWING STROKES To release tension in the neck, support the front of the head with your left hand and use the side of your right hand to rub backward and forward across the base of the skull in a sawing motion. Try to maintain a firm, even pressure. Then knead the base of the neck by squeezing and releasing the flesh with the fingers and thumbs of alternate hands.

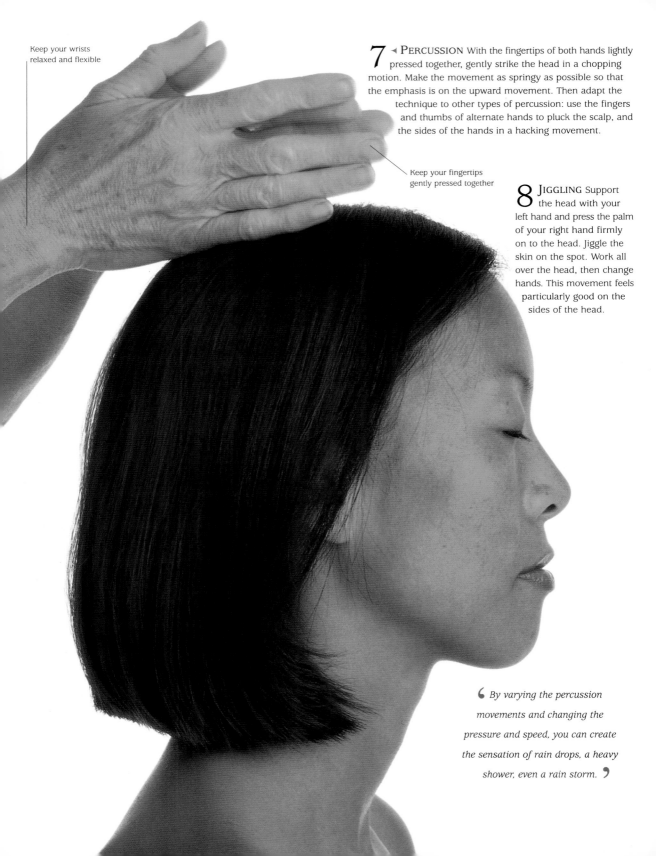

Keep your wrists
relaxed and flexible

7 ◄ PERCUSSION With the fingertips of both hands lightly pressed together, gently strike the head in a chopping motion. Make the movement as springy as possible so that the emphasis is on the upward movement. Then adapt the technique to other types of percussion: use the fingers and thumbs of alternate hands to pluck the scalp, and the sides of the hands in a hacking movement.

Keep your fingertips
gently pressed together

8 JIGGLING Support the head with your left hand and press the palm of your right hand firmly on to the head. Jiggle the skin on the spot. Work all over the head, then change hands. This movement feels particularly good on the sides of the head.

❝ By varying the percussion
movements and changing the
pressure and speed, you can create
the sensation of rain drops, a heavy
shower, even a rain storm. ❞

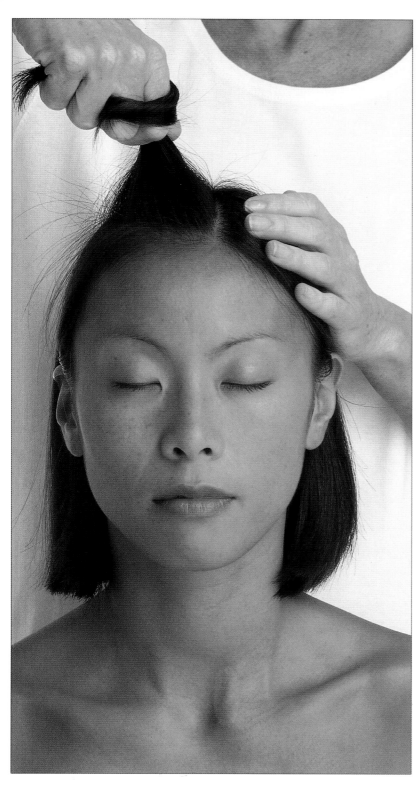

9 ◄ **GENTLE HAIR PULLS** Rest your left hand on the head and with your right, clasp a handful of hair at the roots and twist it around your fingers. Gently pull the hair, hold for a few seconds, then release and repeat with the left hand. Continue pulling and releasing the hair with alternate hands. This movement feels heavenly when done well and quite the opposite if done badly.

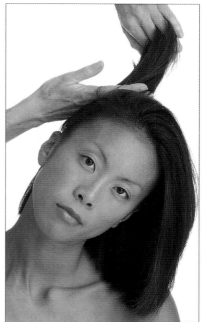

10 ▲ **COMBING** To finish the massage, stroke the fingers of alternate hands gently through the hair, taking care not to pull the hair. Try to make this movement as flowing as possible. Then stroke the fingertips of both hands as lightly as a feather all over the head.

PRACTICE TIPS

To understand the full impact of each technique in this massage, try the sequence on yourself. You may have to adapt some of the steps, but it will help you to master the range of movements.

✦

The pressure techniques in steps 1–3 can also be practiced when applying shampoo or conditioner to the hair.

SHIATSU

SHIATSU, literally translated as "finger pressure," evolved in Japan, and has its origins in traditional Chinese medicine. It is based on the Eastern principle that energy of life (*ki* in Japanese, *qi* in Chinese) flows through longitudinal meridians in the body. The aim is to apply pressure along these meridians, usually with the thumbs or the heels of the hands, to influence the flow of *ki* and maintain harmony and good health. Shiatsu is usually performed through the clothes.

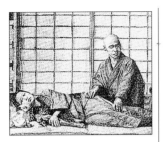

THIS 19TH-CENTURY ENGRAVING ILLUSTRATES THE TRADITIONAL MASSAGE PRACTICE OF *ANMA*, A PRECURSOR TO SHIATSU IN JAPAN.

The pressure of the hands causes the springs of life to flow.

TOKUJIRO NAMIKOSHI,
SHIATSU MASTER, 1972

KEY PRINCIPLES

Like Chinese massage (*see pages 78–81*), shiatsu is based on the theory of meridians. Applying pressure along these meridians is said to influence the flow of *ki*, dispersing energy from where there is an excess of *ki* (*jitsu*) and replenishing areas that are depleted (*kyo*). This is said to re-establish balance and harmony in a person, and so remedy ill health. Some practitioners work on whole meridians while others focus more on specific shiatsu points. There are about 600 points arranged symmetrically on the body.

MAIN SHIATSU POINTS
This schematic illustration shows some of the shiatsu points that are most commonly used.

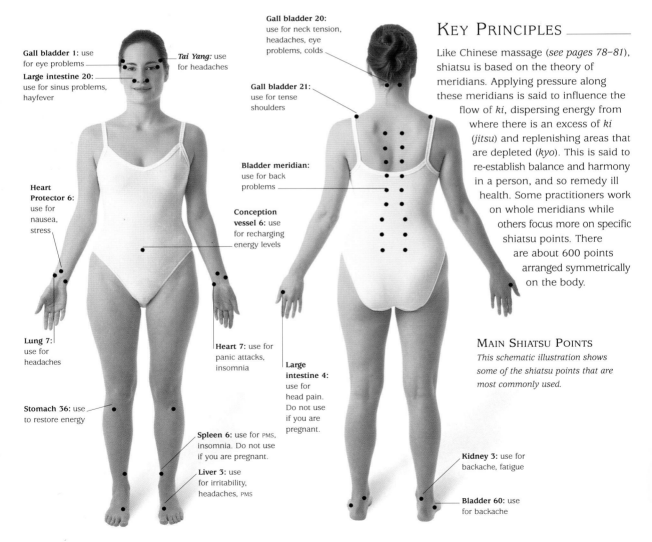

Gall bladder 1: use for eye problems

Large intestine 20: use for sinus problems, hayfever

Tai Yang: use for headaches

Gall bladder 20: use for neck tension, headaches, eye problems, colds

Gall bladder 21: use for tense shoulders

Heart Protector 6: use for nausea, stress

Bladder meridian: use for back problems

Conception vessel 6: use for recharging energy levels

Lung 7: use for headaches

Heart 7: use for panic attacks, insomnia

Large intestine 4: use for head pain. Do not use if you are pregnant.

Stomach 36: use to restore energy

Spleen 6: use for PMS, insomnia. Do not use if you are pregnant.

Liver 3: use for irritability, headaches, PMS

Kidney 3: use for backache, fatigue

Bladder 60: use for backache

PRACTICING SHIATSU

Shiatsu is usually performed on the floor, and it is essential that you use your body weight correctly to apply pressure. Do not prod the skin, but relax with your arms straight, and lean slowly with your body weight. In this way, you can apply very deep pressure without causing pain. Hold the pressure for about five seconds, so that you have time to tune into your partner's body, and so that your partner becomes aware of their own body and relaxes.

The supporting, or "mother," hand is an important concept in shiatsu, and means that one hand is active while the other is receptive and "listens" to the body, encouraging a flow of *ki*. Try to establish a rhythm and work slowly, so that you stay still for a while with each pressure. You can use shiatsu pressures on their own or within another massage sequence.

PRACTICE TIPS

Although a knowledge of the meridians is obviously helpful in shiatsu, you can discover the appropriate places to apply pressure by exploring your partner's body with your hands. Meridians are usually longitudinal lines, so glide your thumb along the limbs, abdomen, and back, and feel for indentations, or points, that seem to "want" to be pressed. Most points give a radiating sensation when pressed, rather like a dull, but pleasurable, ache.

◆

To learn how to relax your body weight on to your hands, spend about five minutes crawling on the floor on your hands and knees.

BACK OF BODY

1 BACK Place the heels of your hands on either side of the spine toward the top of the back, and relax your fingers. Swing your hips forward and lean your body weight on to your partner's back. Hold for about five seconds, then sit back, glide your hands a little further down the back and repeat the pressures. Work down to the hips, then return to the starting position and use your thumbs to apply pressures down the back in the same way.

2 HIPS To work on the hips, you may find it comfortable to kneel astride your partner's legs. With the heels of your hands, apply pressures to the soft, hollow areas in the sacrum, at the base of the spine, moving your hips forward when you lean into a pressure. Work down to the middle of the buttocks, then repeat the pressures with your thumbs.

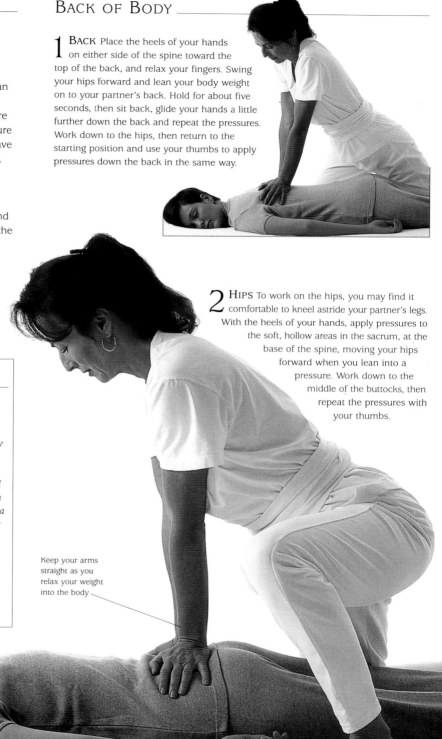

Keep your arms straight as you relax your weight into the body

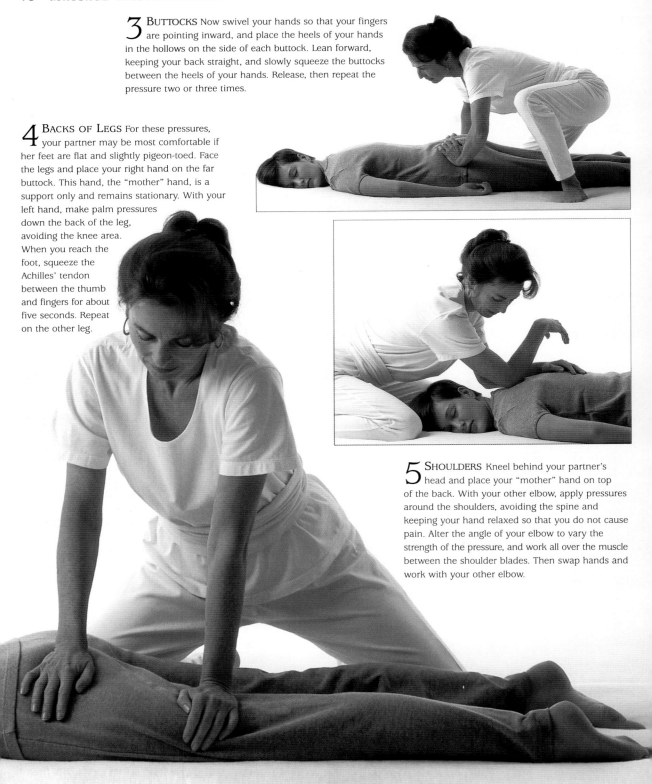

3 BUTTOCKS Now swivel your hands so that your fingers are pointing inward, and place the heels of your hands in the hollows on the side of each buttock. Lean forward, keeping your back straight, and slowly squeeze the buttocks between the heels of your hands. Release, then repeat the pressure two or three times.

4 BACKS OF LEGS For these pressures, your partner may be most comfortable if her feet are flat and slightly pigeon-toed. Face the legs and place your right hand on the far buttock. This hand, the "mother" hand, is a support only and remains stationary. With your left hand, make palm pressures down the back of the leg, avoiding the knee area. When you reach the foot, squeeze the Achilles' tendon between the thumb and fingers for about five seconds. Repeat on the other leg.

5 SHOULDERS Kneel behind your partner's head and place your "mother" hand on top of the back. With your other elbow, apply pressures around the shoulders, avoiding the spine and keeping your hand relaxed so that you do not cause pain. Alter the angle of your elbow to vary the strength of the pressure, and work all over the muscle between the shoulder blades. Then swap hands and work with your other elbow.

FRONT OF BODY

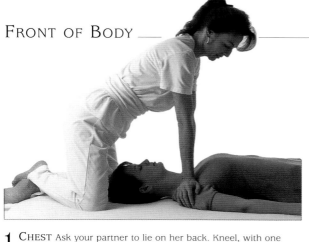

2 FACE Still kneeling behind your partner's head, make thumb pressures all over her forehead and along the eyebrows. Then place your thumbs in the hollows just to the side of each nostril and make a series of pressures under the cheekbones. This helps to clear the sinuses.

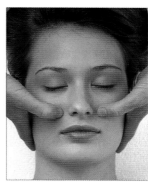

1 CHEST Ask your partner to lie on her back. Kneel, with one knee on either side of her head, and place the heels of your hands in the hollows between the collar bone and shoulder joints, with your fingers facing outward. Bring your hips forward and lean into your partner's shoulders for a few seconds. Then make palm pressures across the chest to the sides of the body, followed by gentle thumb pressures between the ribs. Work down the chest, avoiding the breast tissue.

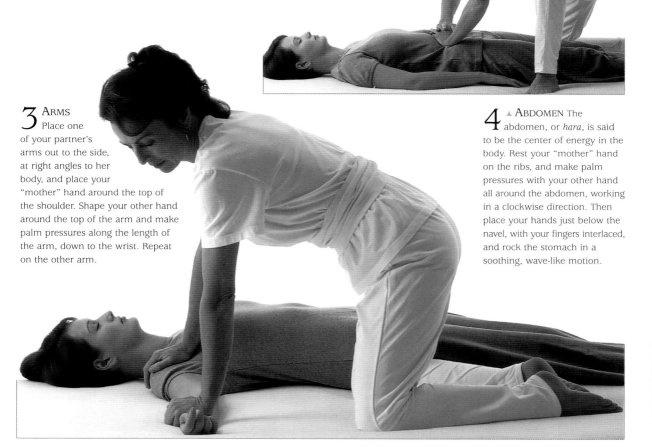

3 ARMS Place one of your partner's arms out to the side, at right angles to her body, and place your "mother" hand around the top of the shoulder. Shape your other hand around the top of the arm and make palm pressures along the length of the arm, down to the wrist. Repeat on the other arm.

4 ▲ ABDOMEN The abdomen, or *hara*, is said to be the center of energy in the body. Rest your "mother" hand on the ribs, and make palm pressures with your other hand all around the abdomen, working in a clockwise direction. Then place your hands just below the navel, with your fingers interlaced, and rock the stomach in a soothing, wave-like motion.

REFLEXOLOGY

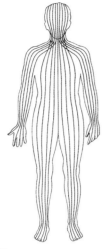

REFLEXOLOGY IS BASED on the theory that applying pressure to specific areas on the feet and, less commonly, on the hands and ears can affect internal organs and body systems, and therefore promote good health. It evolved from the work of Dr. William H. Fitzgerald, a US ear, nose, and throat surgeon, who was interested in the theory of energy lines, or meridians (*see page 78*), and developed "zone therapy" (*see below*) in around 1913. A reflexology treatment tends to be extremely relaxing; not only do most people enjoy having their feet massaged, but stimulating the extensive nerve endings in the feet is beneficial in itself and can have profound effects throughout the body. The sequence opposite is a simple reflexology treatment.

THE ZONES
According to Dr. Fitzgerald's zone therapy, the whole body can be divided into longitudinal zones, or energy channels, that run through the whole body, terminating in the feet and hands. Any part of the body can be stimulated by working on the reflex area of the foot in the same zone.

REFLEX POINTS ON THE FEET

The theory of energy zones was developed further by Dr. Fitzgerald's followers, including Eunice Ingram, who produced charts in the 1930s that "mapped" the soles, sides, and tops of the feet to indicate the locations of reflex points for every part of the body.

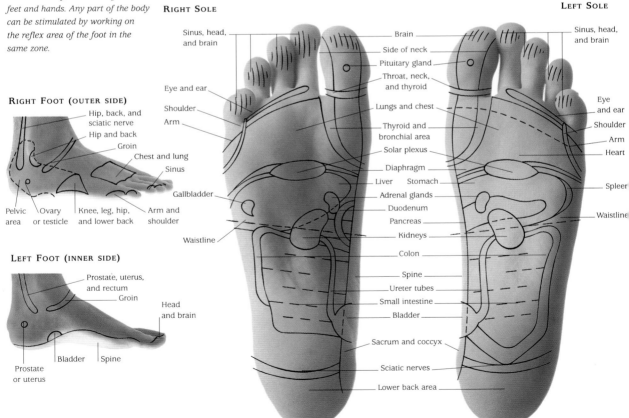

RIGHT FOOT (OUTER SIDE)
- Hip, back, and sciatic nerve
- Hip and back
- Groin
- Chest and lung
- Sinus
- Gallbladder
- Pelvic area
- Ovary or testicle
- Knee, leg, hip, and lower back
- Arm and shoulder
- Waistline
- Eye and ear
- Shoulder
- Arm

LEFT FOOT (INNER SIDE)
- Prostate, uterus, and rectum
- Groin
- Head and brain
- Prostate or uterus
- Bladder
- Spine

RIGHT SOLE
- Sinus, head, and brain
- Eye and ear
- Shoulder
- Arm
- Gallbladder
- Waistline

Brain
Side of neck
Pituitary gland
Throat, neck, and thyroid
- Lungs and chest
- Thyroid and bronchial area
- Solar plexus
- Diaphragm
- Liver   Stomach
- Adrenal glands
- Duodenum
- Pancreas
- Kidneys
- Colon
- Spine
- Ureter tubes
- Small intestine
- Bladder
- Sacrum and coccyx
- Sciatic nerves
- Lower back area

LEFT SOLE
- Sinus, head, and brain
- Eye and ear
- Shoulder
- Arm
- Heart
- Spleen
- Waistline

PRACTICING REFLEXOLOGY

In reflexology, pressure is applied with the thumb or forefinger. You either use a static pressure or a "walking" technique, when a digit is bent and straightened to move it forward. Support the foot throughout, with the other hand as near as possible to the area you are working on. If an area is sensitive, focus on the tender spot until the pain subsides, but always stay within your partner's pain threshold. Work systematically on one foot and then on the other. Avoid using oil, since this makes your fingers slip.

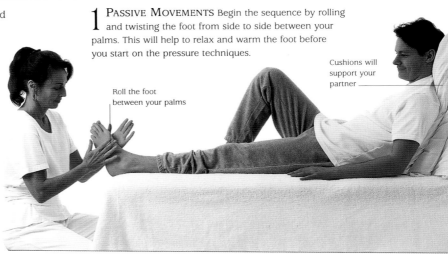

1 PASSIVE MOVEMENTS Begin the sequence by rolling and twisting the foot from side to side between your palms. This will help to relax and warm the foot before you start on the pressure techniques.

Cushions will support your partner

Roll the foot between your palms

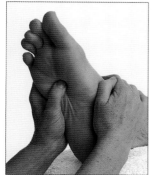

2 DIAPHRAGM AREA Support the top of the foot with your right hand and walk the thumb of your left hand along the diaphragm line, just under the ball of the foot.

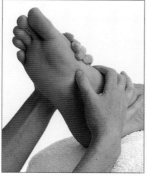

3 SPINAL AREA Use the thumb to apply static or walking pressures from the heel of the foot to the big toe, while your other hand supports the top of the foot.

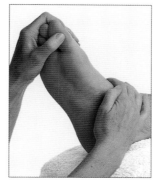

4 HEAD Work up each toe in turn, starting with the little toe and finishing with the big toe. Use your fingers to support the toes and your other hand to support the top of the foot.

5 CHEST AREA Now work between the tendons on the top of the foot. Make a series of pressures along each furrow in turn from the bases of the toes to the ankle.

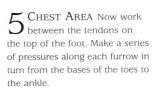

6 DIGESTIVE SYSTEM Apply pressures in diagonal lines from the waistline to the diaphragm line, then from the heel to the waistline.

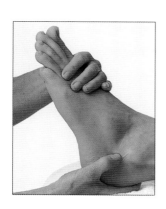

7 REPRODUCTIVE ORGANS & BACK Support the foot firmly and make pressures all around the ankle with your thumb. This area may be quite tender. Then work all over the heel to prevent or treat lower back pain. Finish by stroking the foot gently from the ankle to the toes.

SELF-TREATMENT

Reflexology is very relaxing and is often used to treat stress-related conditions. It is possible to give yourself an effective treatment by exploring the foot with static and walking pressures. Adapt the above sequence, paying extra attention to tender or sensitive areas.

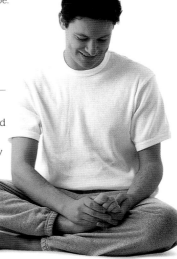

SARAWAK MASSAGE

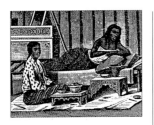

IN THIS 19TH-CENTURY ILLUSTRATION OF AN INDONESIAN LONGHOUSE, THE SCENE IS SET FOR A SLOW, RELAXING MASSAGE.

THE MASSAGE TECHNIQUES that I was taught in Sarawak reflect the fascinating variety of peoples and cultures there – Malay, Chinese, Indian, and Dyak. It was in Sarawak that I learned how versatile kneading could be: strong and energetic, gentle and soporific, or fluid and rhythmic like the beautiful traditional dancing there. The sequence below is slow and methodical, designed to send waves of relaxation through the body.

❛ The experience of a Sarawak massage can be summed up in the Malay word for thank-you, terimakasi, which my masseuse in Kuching told me meant "I have received your love". ❜

1 CALMING STROKES Sit at your partner's head and place one hand on either side of the spine. Stroke very slowly down to the small of the back, leaning into the movement. Repeat at least six times. This downward stroke is incredibly soothing.

2 ◄ RHYTHMIC KNEADING Now face across the body and start to knead the top of the far shoulder with soft hands. As you push the flesh from hand to hand, count "and one, and two, and three" and so on in your head, so that the movement is really rhythmic. On "five," move your hands a little further down the side of the body and repeat. Continue down to the hips in the same way, then return to the start and repeat the sequence three times. Now knead the side of the body nearest to you, or change sides if you prefer, and work again in three rows.

3 STRETCHES Cross your arms, placing one hand on the hip and the other on the opposite shoulder. Lean forward, keeping your arms straight, to stretch the back. Circle around the hip and shoulder, then glide your hands past each other, and repeat on the other shoulder and hip.

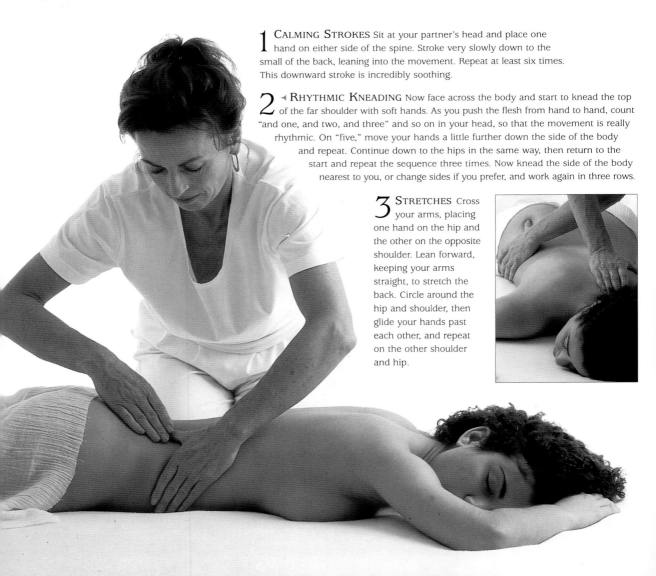

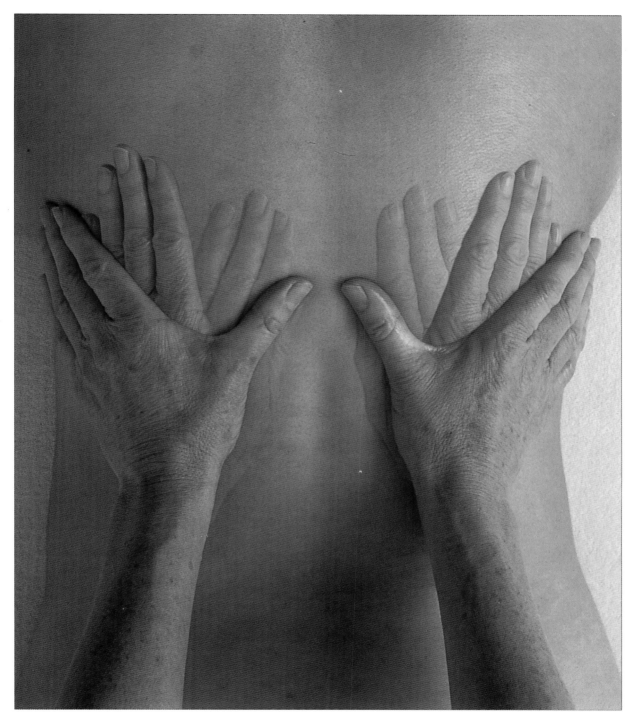

4 SARAWAK SWAY This movement is a variation on the theme of kneading. Place your thumbs on either side of the spine, at the top of the back, molding your fingers around the body. Circle the fingers of both hands in toward the spine. Then stroke your hands down the back a little and fan your fingers up and around again in the same way. Continue to work down the back in a smooth and unbroken movement, counting in your head so that you maintain a steady rhythm.

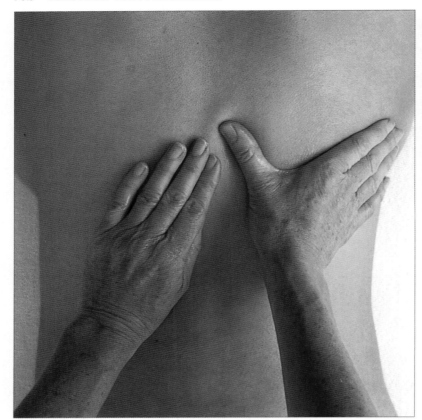

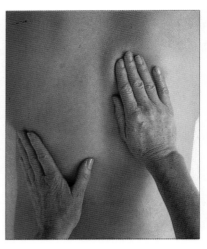

5 SARAWAK SWAY WITH ALTERNATE HANDS Now repeat step 4 but with alternate hands. Begin by circling the fingers of your left hand in toward the spine (*see left*), then follow immediately with the fingers of your right hand as your left hand slides down the back and repeats the stroke (*see above*). The aim is to achieve a fluid, wave-like movement down the back, with the fingers of one hand after the other circling up and around toward the spine. Glide up the back and repeat three times.

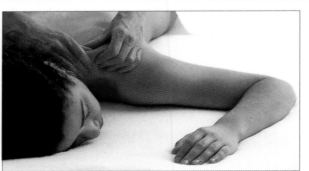

6 ◄ SKIN ROLLING Move to beside your partner's head and place one thumb next to the other on the far shoulder blade. Squeeze the skin with your fingers, then push your thumbs towards your fingertips, rolling the flesh forward. Continue down the side of the body, rolling the skin away from the spine, then stroke the area and repeat on the other side of the body.

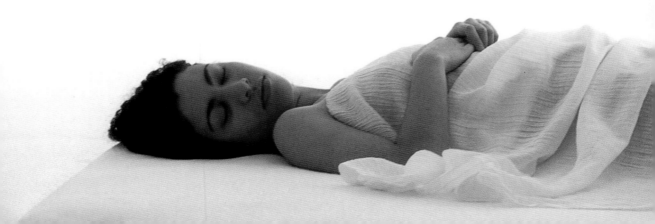

LEGS

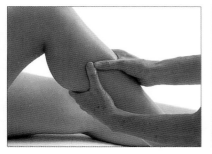

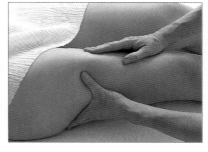

1 CALF STROKES Ask your partner to turn over. Place one hand on top of the foot and the other underneath, and stroke up the foot several times. Then bend the leg and mold your hands around the lower calf, with your thumbs on the outer side. Use your whole hand to stroke slowly up the calf, then glide back and repeat six times.

2 KNEADING Straighten the leg and stroke both hands firmly up the thigh. Then slowly knead the thigh with flat, soft hands. Start on the upper thigh, working up the leg in consecutive rows, so that you cover the whole thigh. As you push the flesh from one hand to the other, count "and one, and two, and three…" up to five, for a steady, soporific rhythm.

3 SARAWAK SWAY WITH ALTERNATE HANDS Place your thumbs on top of the thigh, with your fingers molded around the sides. Circle the fingers of your right hand in toward your thumb while pushing up with your palm. Release the pressure and repeat with the other hand. Work down to the knee with alternate hands circling inward and upward, then stroke up the thigh and repeat the movement six times. You can continue this movement down the calf, working with your thumbs on either side of the bone.

4 ◄ ROLLING STROKES Place your hands on either side of the upper thigh. Start to circle your right hand on the spot, working down and around, then follow with your left hand so that you roll the thigh between your hands. Work down to the knee, then stroke up the leg and repeat. Although you are working down, the pressure is an upward one.

5 HACKING Use the sides of your hands to hack very lightly up and down the thigh, then stroke the whole leg and foot three times. Repeat steps 1–5 on the other leg.

Roll the thigh slowly and firmly between your hands

TURKISH BATHS MASSAGE

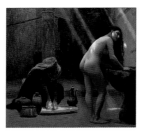

THE MISTY LIGHT AND LAZY AMBIENCE OF A TURKISH BATH IS BROUGHT TO LIFE IN JEAN LEON GEROME'S 19TH-CENTURY PAINTING.

TURKISH BATHS, or *hammams*, have a timeless allure, and the very words conjure up visions of luxury. The first baths, dating back to the time of the ancient Greeks and Romans, had three main purposes: relaxation, refreshment, and the promotion of health. Today, massages are still given with a confidence and strength that is totally invigorating. Here, I have adapted traditional techniques for two uplifting sequences that can be performed with oil or, for authenticity, soap suds.

> *Perfectly massed…you experience a universal content. The blood circulates freely and you feel as if freed from an enormous weight; you enjoy a suppleness and a lightness hitherto unknown.*
>
> CLAUDE SAVARY,
> LETTERS ON EGYPT, 1787

FULL-BODY MASSAGE

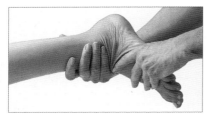

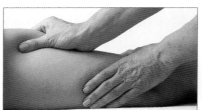

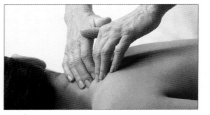

1 FEET Begin by cupping the fingers of both hands under the left foot and use your thumbs to stroke firmly up the sides of the Achilles' tendon and around the ankle bone. Then hold the foot with your left hand, supporting the ankle with your right hand, and slowly rotate it.

2 LEGS Stroke briskly with alternate hands up the left calf to the thigh. Then use your right hand to squeeze and release the thigh in a deep, rhythmic movement as your left hand pushes the flesh toward the right hand. Repeat steps 1–2 on the right foot and leg.

3 BASE OF NECK Stroke up the back. Then, crossing your thumbs for control, make circular finger pressures around the base of the neck, working deep into the muscles. Take care to avoid the spine, and encourage your partner to move her head from side to side for comfort.

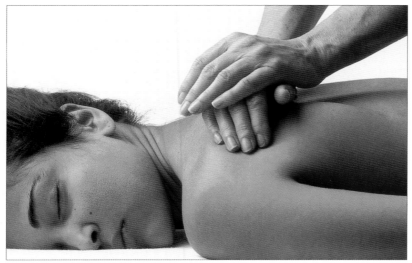

4 SHOULDERS Place one hand on the other and use the heels of your hands to apply circular pressures around each shoulder blade. Lean your body into the stroke to work deeply into the muscle.

PRACTICE TIPS

Turkish massage requires strong, confident hands. Repeatedly squeeze and release a small rubber ball in one hand then the other to gain strength and flexibility in your hands (see also page 13).

◆

When applying pressure, keep your back and arms straight, and lean into the stroke.

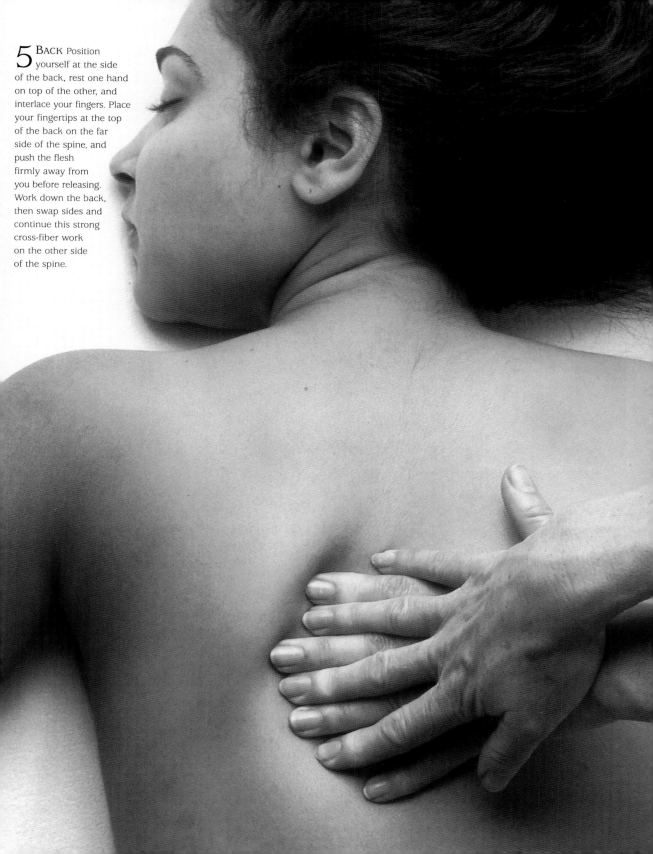

5 BACK Position
yourself at the side
of the back, rest one hand
on top of the other, and
interlace your fingers. Place
your fingertips at the top
of the back on the far
side of the spine, and
push the flesh
firmly away from
you before releasing.
Work down the back,
then swap sides and
continue this strong
cross-fiber work
on the other side
of the spine.

TURKISH MASSAGE WITH SOAP SUDS

Soap suds greatly enhance the effect of a Turkish bath massage sequence by encouraging the hands to slip and slide with depth and energy over the skin. The following routine is designed to give the arms, shoulders, and neck a thorough workout. It is best if the massage takes place with your partner seated, either on a stool with some towels laid on the floor, or in a bath – the more you can emulate a Turkish bath setting the better. Move around your partner as you work, kneeling or squatting by her side when necessary. When working on the face, it is best if your partner lies down and you sit beside her.

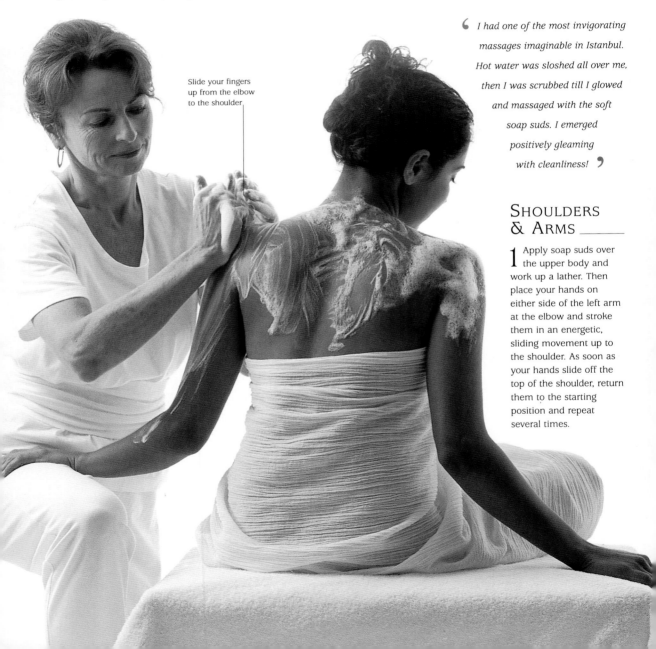

Slide your fingers up from the elbow to the shoulder

6 *I had one of the most invigorating massages imaginable in Istanbul. Hot water was sloshed all over me, then I was scrubbed till I glowed and massaged with the soft soap suds. I emerged positively gleaming with cleanliness!* 9

SHOULDERS & ARMS

1 Apply soap suds over the upper body and work up a lather. Then place your hands on either side of the left arm at the elbow and stroke them in an energetic, sliding movement up to the shoulder. As soon as your hands slide off the top of the shoulder, return them to the starting position and repeat several times.

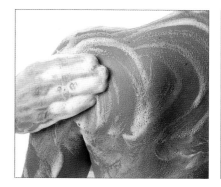

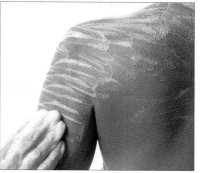

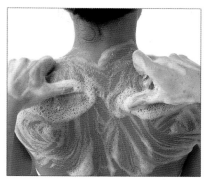

2 Support the front of the left shoulder with your left hand and knead the upper arm and top of the shoulder with your right hand. Use the whole hand to lift and release as much flesh as possible, using a rhythmic, scooping motion.

3 Still supporting the area, zig-zag down the arm with the fingertips of your right hand. Then hold the wrist with your left hand and slowly pull your right hand down the arm, squeezing the flesh as you go. Repeat steps 1–3 on the right arm.

4 Make both your hands into loose fists. Apply slow, circular pressures, rolling your knuckles around the shoulders and on the back of the neck, and using your thumbs for support if you wish. Take care to avoid the spine.

NECK & BACK

1 Use the thumbs and fingers of alternate hands to knead the back of the neck on either side of the spine.

2 ▶ Make slow, circular pressures up the back and neck with your thumbs. The soap will encourage your fingers to slide over the skin without creating friction.

FACE

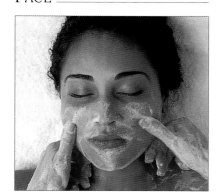

1 ▲ Ask your partner to lie down, and apply soap to her face. Stroke your thumbs firmly along the jaw, then under the cheekbones, stroking out to the temples.

2 Use your fingers to make energetic spirals all over the face, paying attention to the sides of the face and jaw, where tension is often stored.

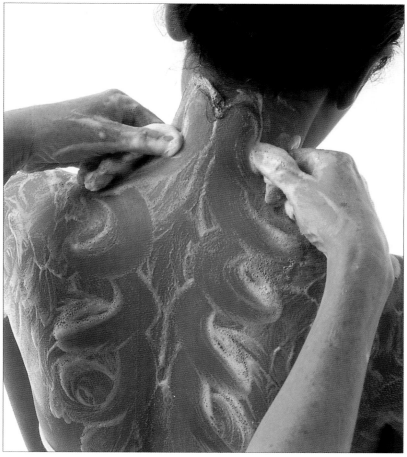

MOROCCAN MASSAGE

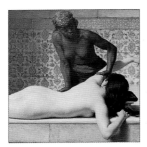

A TYPICAL HAMMAM MASSAGE TAKES PLACE ON A MARBLE SLAB, AS SHOWN HERE IN EDOUARD DESAT-PONSON'S 1883 PAINTING.

IN MOROCCO, as in much of North Africa, massage is offered at the local baths, or *hammams*, and is also given by midwives. The full-body massage that I was taught can be performed in just 15 minutes, and consists mainly of fast stroking. The vigor of the strokes forces the body and mind to let go, and this kind of massage is useful for revitalizing rushed, hyperactive people. You will need a fair amount of energy to do the massage but with practice you will be able to relax into its rhythm.

❛ Let me travel the world to its very end, to many lands, that I might find someone, who can soothe and revive me with their hands. ❜

ATTRIBUTED TO IBN BATUTA, THE 14TH CENTURY ARABIAN TRAVELLER

FRONT OF BODY

1 ABDOMEN Place your hands on the abdomen and stroke one after the other in a large circle around the navel, working in a clockwise direction. As your arms cross, lift one hand over the other and place it on the abdomen to start again. Work firmly and with confidence.

2 ▸ CHEST Position yourself at your partner's head and stroke both hands firmly down the sternum. Then glide back up the sides and pull up at the armpits to create a stretch. Repeat several times.

3 ▾ ARMS Hold your partner's elbow with one hand and stroke your other hand repeatedly and energetically up to the top of the arm, around the shoulder, and back to the elbow. Then support the wrist with one hand and stroke up the forearm in a similar way. Repeat on the other arm.

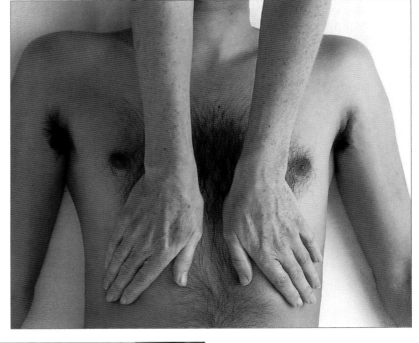

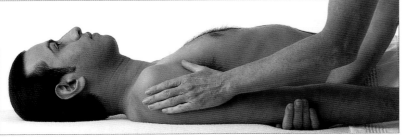

4 LEGS Stroke firmly and briskly up the thigh with one hand after the other. When you reach the top of the leg, glide down the sides. Then stroke the knuckles of alternate hands up the thigh, gliding back with your palms. Repeat several times, then move on to the calf. Place one hand behind the other on the lower calf and use the "V" of your hands to stroke up to the knees. Repeat on the other leg.

BACK OF BODY

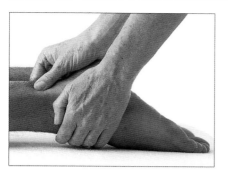
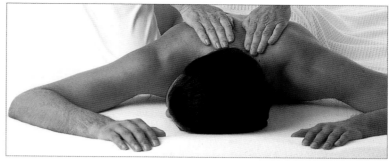

1 LEGS Ask your partner to turn over. Stroke up the left leg a few times and follow by lightly kneading the leg, squeezing and pushing the flesh from one hand to the other. Then support the foot with one hand and use the fingers and thumb of your other hand to stroke firmly and repeatedly up and around either side of the Achilles' tendon. Repeat on the right leg.

2 SHOULDERS Place your hands on either side of the spine at the base of the neck. Pull back with your body weight and circle around and around the fleshy area, where we all hold so much tension. Repeat several times, then move on to the back. Place your hands on either side of the spine at the lower back and stroke firmly up the back. As you reach the ribs, fan your hands out, shaping them around the body, then glide down the sides. Repeat several times, fanning your hands out further up the back each time.

Use the weight of your body to achieve depth and rhythm

3 ▶ BACK Place your right hand at the base of the back and stroke the knuckles of your left hand firmly up one side of the spine. When you reach the top of the back, glide back with your left palm and begin to stroke the knuckles of your right hand up the other side of the spine. Continue for a while, aiming for a rhythmic, energetic movement.

4 HIPS Place your hands on either side of the spine at the sacrum and fan out to the waist in a firm, definite stroke. Then glide smoothly down the sides of the body, pulling up at the buttocks to return to the starting position. Repeat this step at least six times.

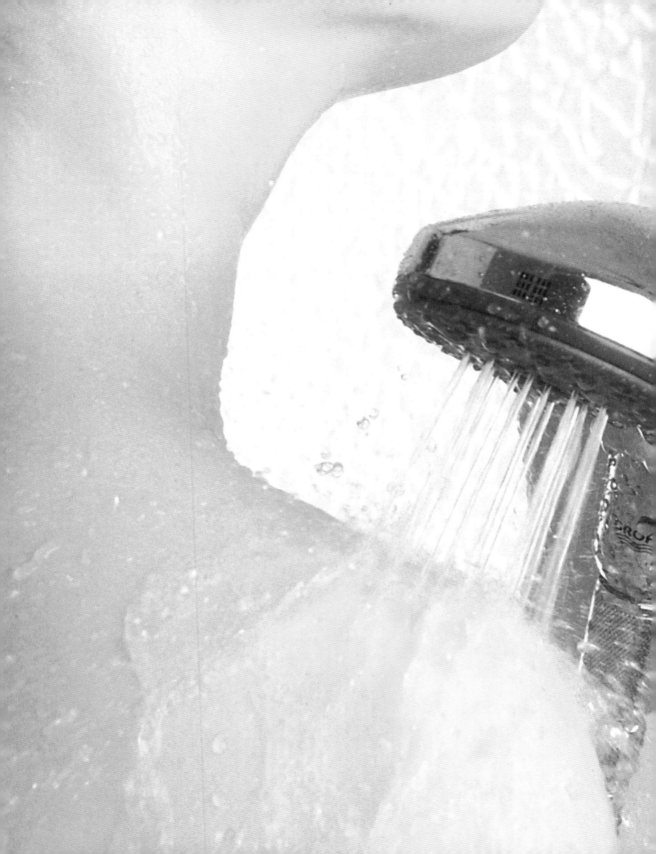

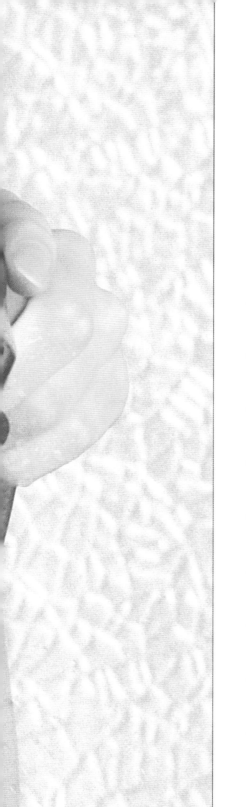

MASSAGE TO
BEAUTIFY

BEAUTY IS TRUER AND DEEPER THAN WE NORMALLY

ALLOW, AND IT ARISES FROM HEALTH IN MIND AND BODY.

BY STIMULATING THE CIRCULATION, NOURISHING THE

SKIN, RELAXING THE MUSCLES, AND CALMING THE MIND,

MASSAGE AND THE USE OF ESSENTIAL OILS HELPS YOU TO

ACHIEVE GLOWING SKIN, SHINING EYES, A RELAXED BODY,

AND AN OPTIMISTIC SPIRIT. MASSAGE CAN THEREFORE

BE A TRULY COMPREHENSIVE BEAUTY TREATMENT THAT

KEEPS YOU LOOKING YOUNG AND FEELING BEAUTIFUL.

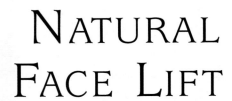

NATURAL FACE LIFT

Face massage is the most relaxing and, I believe, the most beneficial of all massage. Due to the vast number of nerve receptors in the face, massage here has a particularly powerful effect on the nervous system, and affects the whole body (*see page 161*). In just ten minutes it can leave the receiver looking ten years younger and feeling stress-free. Begin by gently stroking the whole face, then focus on the muscles of expression, imagining that you are sculpting the face and giving a face lift with your hands.

THE FACIAL MUSCLES

The muscles in the face, unlike those in the rest of the body, are inserted into the skin, and therefore directly affect the way we look. Our moods and emotions are expressed in our faces, and it is the face that we look at to see how someone is feeling. Stress and tension can have a detrimental effect on our appearance, tightening the muscles, and leading to a pinched, hard look. Massage relaxes this tension and encourages a softer expression.

As muscular tissue in the face becomes weaker with age, fine lines may appear around the mouth, eyes, and forehead. Face massage helps to delay the ageing process by boosting circulation, improving the tone of the muscles, and leaving the recipient radiant and glowing with health.

> *A blemish in the soul cannot be corrected in the face, but a blemish in the face, if corrected, can refresh the soul.*
>
> JEAN COCTEAU (1889–1963)

GENTLE FACIAL OIL BLEND

Essential oils *2 drops each chamomile and geranium oil*
Carrier oil *2 tsp (10 ml) sweet almond oil*

✦

Blend the oils in a bottle (*see pages 14–15*).

SOOTHING, SUPERFICIAL STROKES

When massaging the face, your touch needs to be gentle yet confident. The movements can be deep but should never be heavy; practice on yourself first. Apply the oil (*see recipe, left*) with soft, molding hands.

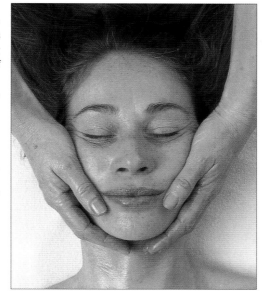

1 ▶ Stroke both hands up the neck to the chin and then from the chin to the ears. Pause, then glide back down to the chin and stroke up to beside the nose. Pause again, stroke under the cheekbones to the temples, then glide back and stroke up the bridge of the nose and across the forehead to the temples. The movement should be gentle and flowing.

2 Rest your thumbs on the bridge of the nose, or the "third eye," and stroke your fingers around the chin and jaw and up to the temples. Use your body weight to lean into the stroke. Repeat several times.

3 Stroke both hands up the neck, and as you reach the jaw, swivel your hands and interlock your fingers. Then stroke each hand out along the jaw and up to the temples. Interlock your fingers again so that the heels of your hands press into the temples, then stroke your fingers out across the forehead. Repeat several times.

❛ *If your partner wears contact lenses, make sure she removes them before starting the massage.* ❜

CHEST & NECK

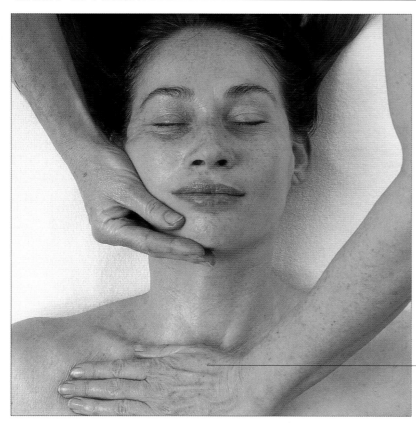

Sweep one hand across the chest as the other strokes around the jaw

1 ◀ Rhythmically stroke up one side of the neck, with one hand following the other, at least ten times. Then continue on the other side by gliding your top hand around the jaw and stroking your bottom hand across the chest. Now stroke up this side of the neck in the same way. Repeat several times, so that one hand strokes around the jaw as the other sweeps across the chest. Aim for a seamless movement.

2 Begin as you did in step 1, by stroking one hand after the other up the side of the neck. Then adapt the movement slightly by stroking your top hand up the side of the face and across the forehead as your lower hand sweeps across the chest and up the neck to meet the top hand at the jaw. Stroke up the side of the neck ten times, then repeat the whole movement, making the sequence as smooth as possible.

JAW & CHIN

1 Lodge your fingers under the chin and use your thumbs to circle along the jaw. Circle one thumb in a clockwise direction and the other in a counterclockwise direction, applying a slight lift as your thumbs circle toward one another.

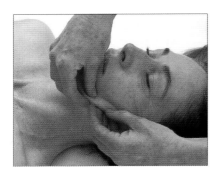

2 Stroke one hand after the other up the left cheek from the chin to the ears a few times. Repeat on the right side. Then extend the stroke so that you circle each hand around the chin before stroking up the cheek. This is a lovely, rhythmic stroke.

4 ◄ Using the fingers and thumbs of alternate hands, knead the jaw, working from the left ear to the chin. Squeeze and release the flesh slowly and gently, then repeat the movement on the right side.

5 ► Finish with knuckling the hands on each cheek to release any jaw tension. Roll your knuckles in a strong, circular motion, rotating your wrists up and out toward the ears as you do so.

3 With your thumbs stabilized on the forehead, apply circular pressures over the chin and jaw with your fingertips. Start gently, then work deeper. Ask your partner to clench her teeth for a moment so that you can locate where there may be tension.

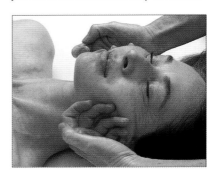

MOUTH & CHEEKS

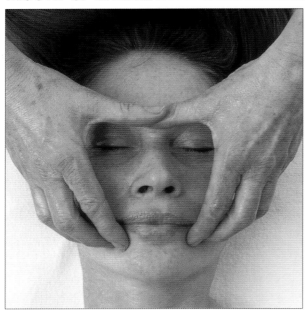

1 Place one thumb on top of the other, and rest them both on the bridge of the nose for support. Gently stroke your ring fingers from the center of the mouth to each corner. Slowly introduce your second fingers, followed by your index fingers. Repeat across the upper lip, then on the lower lip.

2 Keep your hands in the same position and use the tips of your index and second fingers to make circular pressures at the corners of the mouth. Circle in one direction then the other, working slowly and deeply. Then work all around the mouth.

3 Support the right cheek with your right hand and make large circles with your left palm on the left cheek, working in a counterclockwise direction. Then swap sides so that you make circles with your right hand as your left hand remains stationary. Repeat several times, then rotate both hands alternately, applying more pressure on the upward movement.

4 Stroke out to the ears, then use your thumbs and fingertips to squeeze and rotate each ear, working systematically to cover the whole area. This can feel surprisingly soothing.

EYES

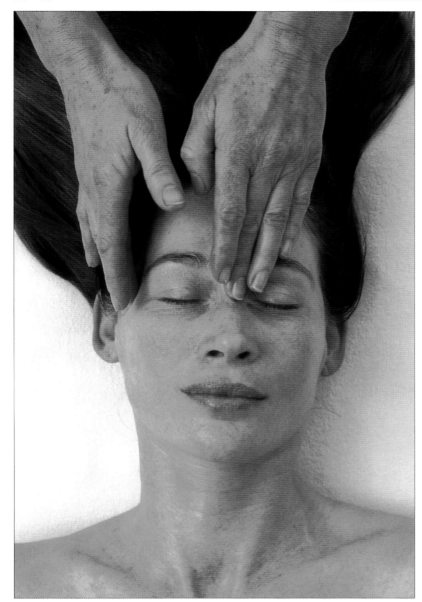

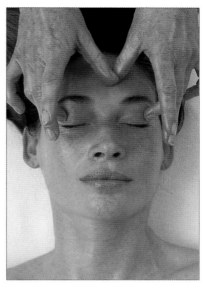

4 Cross the thumbs for stability, and glide your ring fingers very gently over the eyelids from the center to the corners. Then apply gentle, circular pressures at the corners of the eyes, easing away any laughter lines.

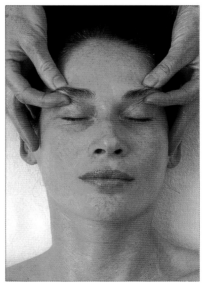

1 Make sure that your partner has removed any contact lenses before starting this sequence. Stroke your index and second fingers firmly over the eyebrows from the nose to the temples, then softly under the eyes back to the nose.

2 Now use your hands alternately, so that one hand strokes over the eyebrow as the other strokes beneath the eye.

3 ▲ Place your second fingers on the corner of each eye. With the second finger of your left hand, stroke under the eye, up and across the bridge of the nose and toward the right eye. When it meets your right hand, stroke it back under the right eye and across the left eyebrow. Repeat this movement with the second finger of your right hand. Try to make these figure-of-eight strokes smooth and soporific.

5 Squeeze the eyebrows at the bridge of the nose between your thumbs and index fingers. Hold for a couple of seconds, then release and squeeze a little further along. Work out to the temples, gently squeezing and releasing the flesh.

FOREHEAD

1 Stroke one hand after the other up the forehead into the hairline. Stroke slowly and hypnotically, making sure that your hands are relaxed. Although this may feel boring for you, the sheer repetitiveness is what feels so relaxing for your partner.

2 Make circular pressures at the temples and all over the forehead. Start with your little fingers, then follow with each of your other fingers, experimenting with the speed, depth, and direction of the circles according to your partner's wishes.

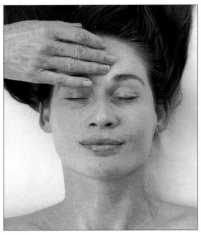

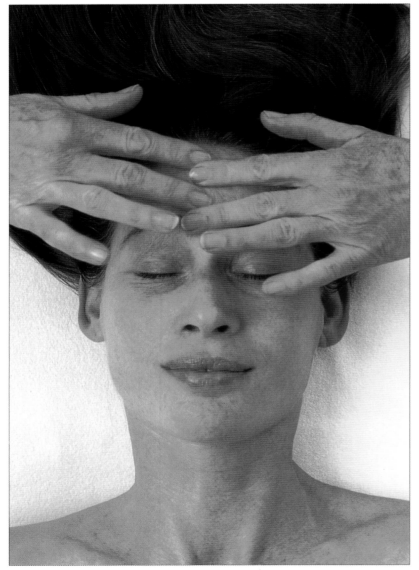

4 ▲ Support the top of the head with one hand and make light, circular strokes at the bridge of the nose with the middle finger of your other hand. Gradually spiral up the center of the forehead with your finger and, when you reach the hairline, stroke your hand in a scooping movement, up into the hair. Return your hand to the starting position and repeat.

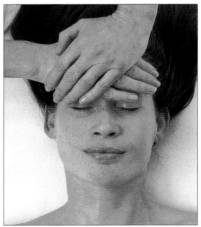

5 To finish the massage, place both your palms on the forehead, one on top of the other, and hold them in place for about a minute. Focus on the rhythm of your partner's breathing. Gradually begin to release the pressure and then lift your hands away as slowly as possible. This relaxing hold should leave your partner feeling incredibly calm and secure.

3 ▲ To combat frown lines, place your hands across the forehead and press firmly with the first two fingers of each hand. Make zig-zagging strokes with your hands moving toward each other. Cover the whole forehead with this soft, scissoring action, varying the speed of the strokes, and concentrating on areas of tension.

TONING TECHNIQUES

Although most of the strokes used on the face are gentle and flowing, fast, staccato movements are also used. These have a wonderfully stimulating and toning effect on the skin, and can be used to add variety to a sequence. Surprisingly, these staccato movements can also be extraordinarily relaxing, obliterating all thought in your massage partner and forcing the mind to rest and the muscles to let go. Practice the following routine on your knee before attempting it on your partner. You will only need a few drops of oil.

1 Using all four fingers of each hand, stroke briskly up the left side of the neck, one hand after the other. Roll your fingers to get a lifting effect at the end of each stroke, then repeat on the right side. Try the same movement under the jaw with your hands facing each other and your elbows out so that you use the pads of your fingers, rather than the tips. Flick away those double chins!

2 ▼ Continue with some energetic drumming. Use the middle fingers of each hand to pat lightly under the chin, once with your left hand, twice with your right. Try to achieve a fast, even tempo.

3 Lean over toward the left side of your partner's face and, with alternate hands, roll one finger after the other up the cheek from the corner of the mouth to the ear in a light, flicking movement. Repeat on the right side.

4 Try the same movement on the forehead. Start just above the eyebrows and, with your hands facing one another, drum the fingers of one hand after the other up the forehead so that you roll the skin towards the hairline. Keep your wrists loose and relaxed for a fast, rhythmic effect.

5 Tap the fingertips of both hands all over the face and forehead, varying the speed and depth of the movement.

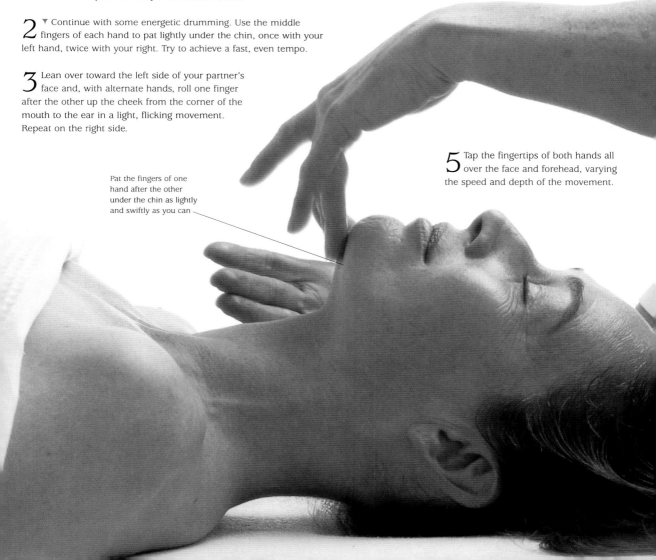

Pat the fingers of one hand after the other under the chin as lightly and swiftly as you can

ANTI-CELLULITE MASSAGE

CELLULITE IS A CONDITION that many women know about, yet medical experts often dismiss it as simply fat. The unsightly "orange-peel" effect caused by dimpled skin can develop on the thighs, hips, and stomach, and is a sad fact of life for a great many women. Women's thighs and stomachs are said to be especially susceptible to fat storage just below the skin. The way in which skin is attached to muscle is rather like the mesh-like structure of a string vest. When fat builds up, it fills the gaps between the skin and the muscle, and this is thought to cause the dimpled appearance associated with cellulite. Whatever cellulite is, self-massage can improve its overall appearance, making it look firmer and smoother. If cellulite is solid and hard, you can use firm movements to soften the area and stimulate circulation; if cellulite feels soft and watery, your movements should be more gentle to encourage lymphatic drainage (see pages 74–77).

TIPS TO COMBAT CELLULITE

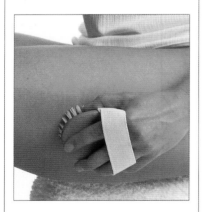

Brush the skin regularly, especially before a bath or shower, with a natural-fiber skin brush or glove. Start at the thigh and work down the leg, using circular upward movements. This helps to stimulate the circulation and lymphatic system (see pages 162–163) and removes dead skin cells.

✦

Drink at least eight glasses of water a day.

✦

Eat a balanced, healthy diet that includes plenty of fresh fruit and vegetables, and avoid too much salt, sugar, or processed food.

ANTI-CELLULITE OIL BLEND

Essential oils *1 drop each rosemary, geranium, and juniper oil*
Carrier oil *2 tsp (10 ml) sunflower oil*
✦
Blend the oils in a bottle (see pages 14–15).

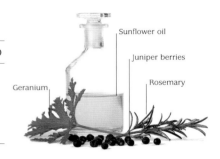

Sunflower oil

Juniper berries

Rosemary

Geranium

THIGH MASSAGE

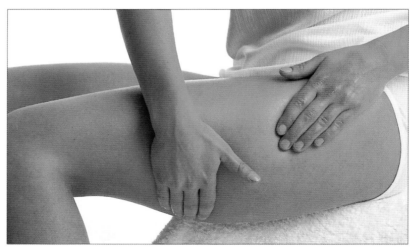

1 Pour some massage oil into one hand and warm it between both palms. Then stroke one hand after the other firmly up the thigh, starting at the knee. Mold your hands to the contours of your leg, and as each hand reaches the top of the thigh, return it to the starting position. Repeat, making sure that you cover the whole thigh.

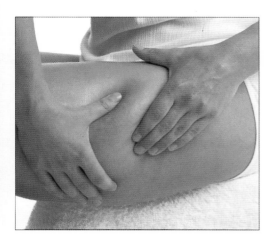

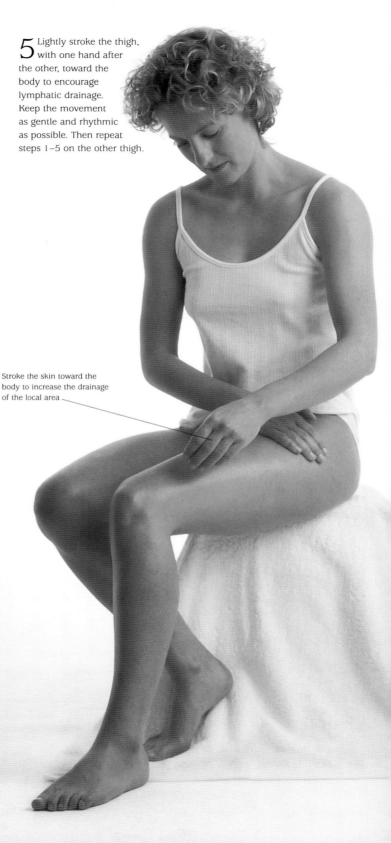

5 Lightly stroke the thigh, with one hand after the other, toward the body to encourage lymphatic drainage. Keep the movement as gentle and rhythmic as possible. Then repeat steps 1–5 on the other thigh.

2 Knead the whole thigh, starting at the knee. Use deep movements to pick up, squeeze, and push the flesh from one hand to the other. You may find it easiest to work in rows along the top, sides, and bottom of the thigh, so that you cover the whole area.

3 Now use the knuckles of each hand to make deep, rotary movements over the thigh. Start at the knee, then work systematically towards the body in the same way as you did in step 2.

Stroke the skin toward the body to increase the drainage of the local area

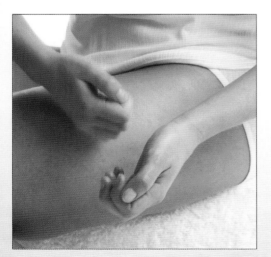

4 Gently pummel the top and outside of your thigh with loose fists. Keep your wrists relaxed to make the movement lively. You may want to reposition your leg slightly so that you can lean right over the area you are working on. This energetic movement stimulates the flow of blood to the surface of the skin.

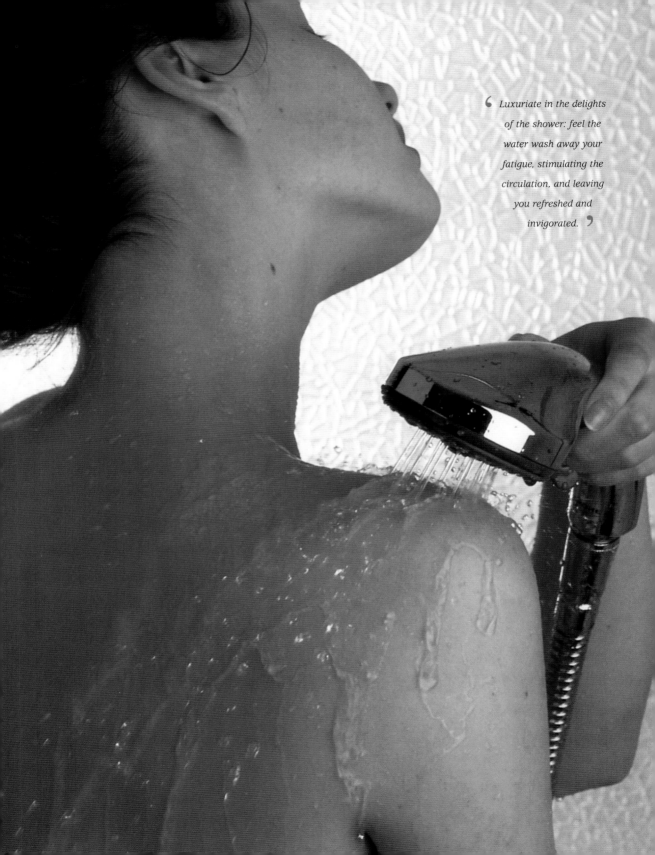

HYDROTHERAPY

Hydrotherapy, or water therapy, techniques make a great addition to massage and can be easily incorporated into a shower or bathtime routine. Water affects the body in different ways according to its temperature. Hot water encourages the muscles to relax by raising the body's temperature; cold water helps to stimulate the circulation and reduce inflammation, and has an invigorating effect on the skin. The sequence below is designed to revitalize the whole body and leave the skin glowing. For maximum benefit, you will need a shower with different flow settings, but any handheld shower should work effectively.

INSTANT INVIGORATION

1 ▶ First remove dead skin with a salt scrub (*see recipe, below*). Stand in the bath or shower and apply the mixture to moist skin. Massage the whole body with circular strokes, paying extra attention to the elbows, knees, and feet. Rinse well.

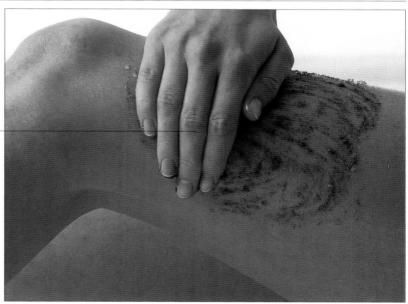

Apply the scrub with circular movements

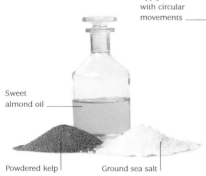

Sweet almond oil

Powdered kelp

Ground sea salt

SALT SCRUB

1 tbsp ground sea salt

1 tbsp powdered kelp

3 tsp (15ml) sweet almond oil

✦

Blend the ingredients in a small bowl.

2 ◀ Switch the shower to hot, and turn it to the strongest setting. Using small, circling movements, massage all around each leg with the shower jet. Then gradually work up the body, spending extra time on areas that feel tense. Massage around the chest, shoulders, and neck, and down each arm. Allow about five minutes in total for the hot shower massage.

3 Repeat the shower massage with cold water, using the same circling movements as before. This alternating of hot and cold water is one of the simplest ways to boost energy levels and will leave you feeling refreshed and invigorated.

4 To complete the routine, dry your skin and massage your whole body with the oil blend (*see right*) using large, circling movements. Orange essential oil has a mildly astringent action on the skin, while frankincense is used to combat dry skin.

Frankincense

EXOTIC OIL BLEND

Essential oils *5 drops each orange and frankincense oil*

Carrier oil *4 tsp (20ml) sweet almond oil*

✦

Blend the oils in a bottle (*see pages 14–15*).

Sweet almond oil

Orange peel

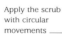

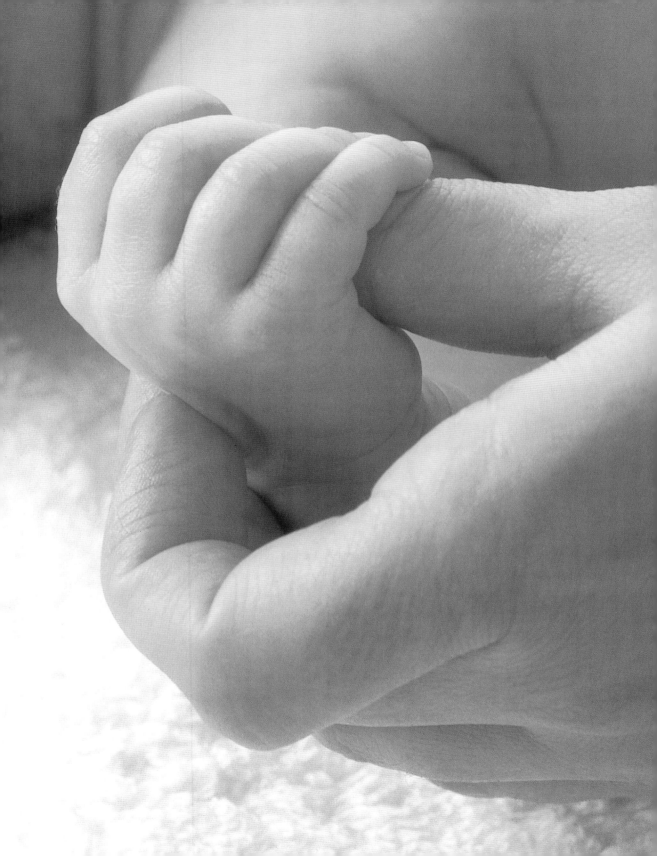

PREGNANCY, BABIES & CHILDREN

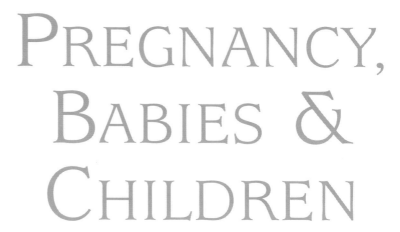

AT ALL STAGES OF PREGNANCY, UP TO AND INCLUDING

THE BIRTH, A MOTHER'S BODY UNDERGOES IMMENSE

UPHEAVALS; MASSAGE CAN BE A POSITIVE BOON THAT

CALMS TENSION AND REDUCES PAIN. A MOTHER'S LOVING,

INSTINCTIVE STROKING CAN EASILY BE DEVELOPED INTO

A MASSAGE, AND RESEARCH SHOWS THAT THIS CAN

ENCOURAGE SLEEP AND BOOST A BABY'S IMMUNE SYSTEM.

AS A CHILD GROWS, THE BENEFITS OF MASSAGE CONTINUE.

MASSAGE FOR PREGNANCY

Massage can be of enormous benefit during pregnancy, helping to soothe jangled nerves and alleviate common complaints such as backache, tension in the shoulders, and aching legs and feet. I massage my clients throughout pregnancy and encourage their partners to do the same. It is a wonderful way for the father to stay truly involved with the pregnancy. Gentle, calming strokes stimulate the circulation without placing extra strain on the heart, and can reduce blood pressure and heart-rate, helping to calm both mother and baby. Spend time making sure that your partner is comfortable; you may want to adapt the positions shown in the following sequences. It is essential that you check with a doctor before using massage in pregnancy.

SOOTHING STROKES

1 ▸ Ask your partner to kneel on the floor with a pile of cushions to lean on. Place both your hands on her lower back, on either side of the spine, and stroke firmly up to the shoulders. Squeeze the tops of the shoulders.

2 Stroke down each arm as far as you can reach, then glide back up the arms and down the sides of the body. Stroke around the hips, over the thighs, down the calves and feet, and around the buttocks to the starting position on the back. Repeat this several times, aiming for a single, unbroken stroke that flows effortlessly over the whole body.

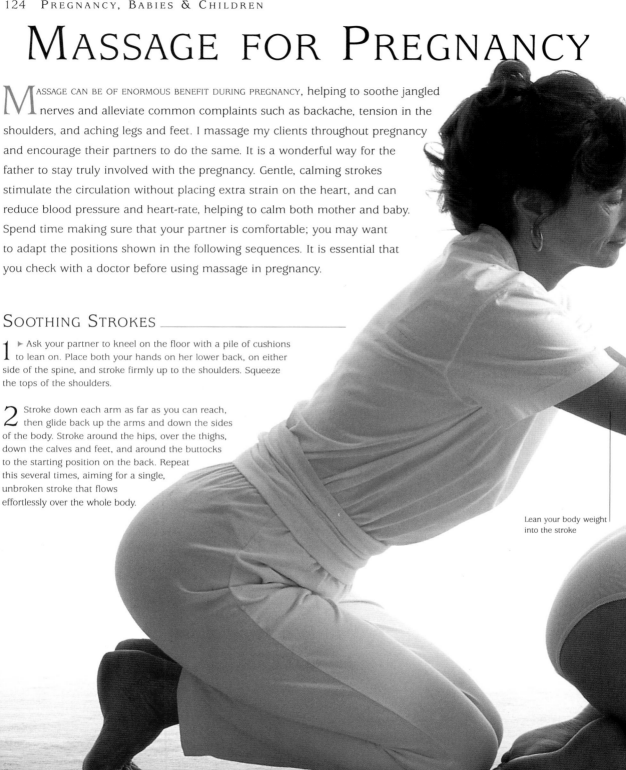

Lean your body weight into the stroke

UPPER BACK RELEASE

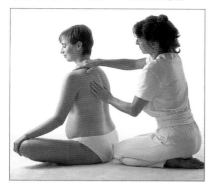
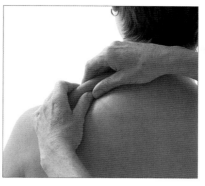
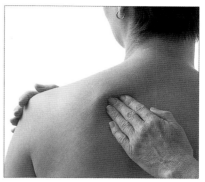

1 For this sequence, your partner may prefer to sit up. Begin with some circle stroking on her left shoulder blade. Stroke one hand after the other in a large circle and, as one hand meets the other wrist, lift it over and complete the circle on the other side, while the other hand continues stroking. Aim for a smooth movement.

2 Knead the top of the left shoulder by rhythmically squeezing and then releasing the flesh with alternate hands. Next, try skin rolling (*see above*), using your thumbs to roll the flesh up the shoulder blade toward your fingers to create a squeeze at the top of the shoulder. This warming action helps to break down tension in the area.

3 Support the front of the body with your right hand and, with the fingertips of your left hand, apply deep, circular pressures along the left shoulder blade, pushing up and under the bone. Finish the massage sequence by stroking your hand gently over the whole area, then repeat steps 1–3 on the right shoulder.

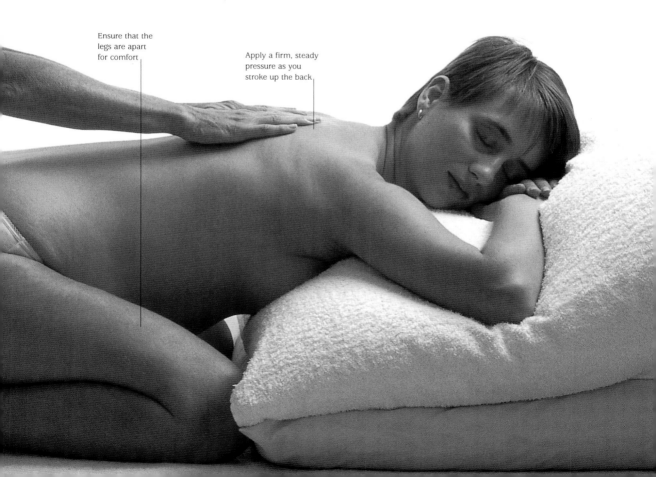

Ensure that the legs are apart for comfort

Apply a firm, steady pressure as you stroke up the back

ABDOMEN MASSAGE

Massaging the stomach with soft, gentle movements is a lovely way to feel close to both mother and child; it can also benefit both of them, as soothing strokes have been reported to calm active, kicking babies. During the first 20 weeks of pregnancy, it is possible to perform the following massage with your partner lying on her back. After this time, the weight of the fetus in this position can constrict circulation, and it is safer, as well as more comfortable, for your partner to lie on her side with her legs bent forward. Place pillows under her head and between her knees to support her.

1 ▶ Side stroking is a particularly effective movement to do during pregnancy, since there is a large surface area to work on. Kneel behind your partner, and stroke one hand after the other very gently up and over the stomach. The hand nearest to your partner's hips can continue the stroke around the lower back before lifting off the skin and repeating the movement.

2 ▼ Now try very light circle stroking. Use both hands to trace a large circle around the abdomen, one hand following the other in a clockwise direction. As your arms cross, lift one hand over the other, making a complete circle with one hand and a half circle with the other. This movement is so superficial that it should feel like little more than a caress. You can also try using one hand to circle the abdomen, gradually making the circle smaller and smaller until you are just circling around the navel.

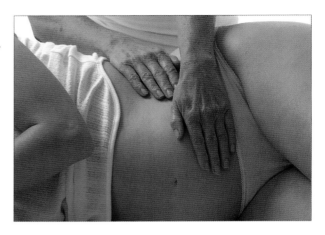

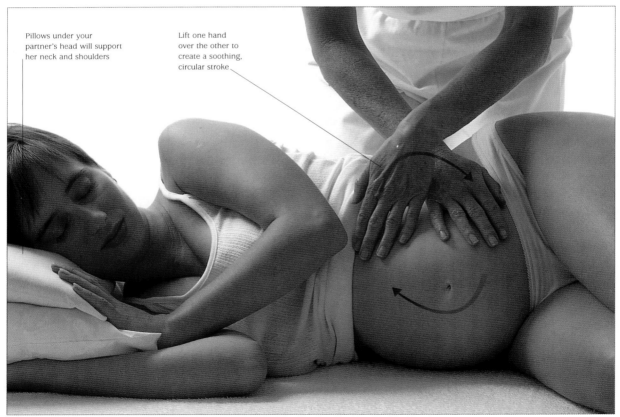

Pillows under your partner's head will support her neck and shoulders

Lift one hand over the other to create a soothing, circular stroke

FOOT MASSAGE

One of the minor ailments that many women complain about during pregnancy is tired, aching feet and ankles. A massage around these areas not only relieves aches and pains but also revitalizes the whole body. Your partner may find it most comfortable to sit in a semi-reclining position propped up with pillows. You can work quite deeply on the feet, but remember to tailor the massage to your partner's needs and desires. Work on one foot then the other.

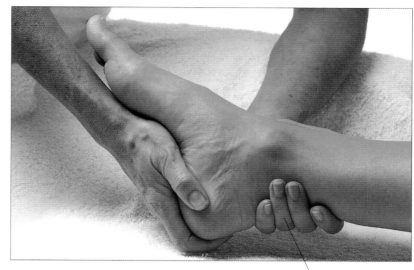

Support the ankle with the fingers of one hand

1 Sandwich the top of your partner's foot between your palms and stroke both hands firmly from the toes toward the body. Glide gently back again, then repeat the same movement several times to accustom your partner to your touch.

2 ▲ Now cup the fingers of one hand under the ankle to support it, and use the thumb of your other hand to stroke deeply all around the heel of the foot.

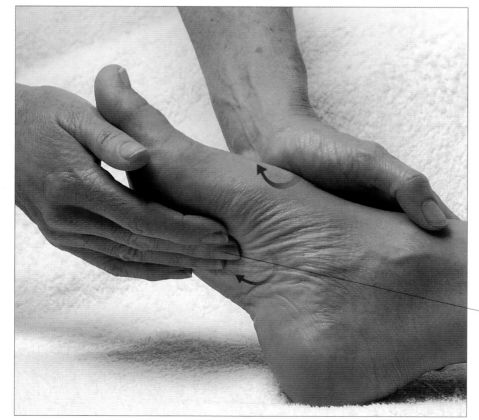

Apply deep, circular pressure with the fingers of the lower hand

3 ◄ Place the heel of one hand on top of the foot, just above the toes, and begin to apply circular pressures, pushing firmly toward the body on the upward stroke. With the fingers of the other hand, make circular pressures on the sole of the foot. Use your hands together to build a strong, steady rhythm. Then squeeze and stroke each toe.

4 Finish the massage by stroking the foot as you did at the beginning. Then, as a final touch, hold the foot between both hands for a few seconds. Release and repeat steps 1–4 on the other foot.

MASSAGE DURING LABOR

M ASSAGING YOUR PARTNER OR FRIEND during childbirth is a positive way to provide reassurance. Overly tense abdominal muscles can delay childbirth, so anything you do to encourage relaxation will be beneficial. As the body relaxes, endorphins, the body's natural pain-killers, are released and stress levels drop. Women react in different ways to labor: some love to be massaged, others suddenly cannot bear to be touched. Always be guided by your partner's needs. Massage can promote relaxation between contractions, as well as alleviate pain during labor. The best position for your partner may be one in which she is leaning forward. This gives the baby room to move into the right position for delivery. Always make sure that the doctor is aware of your intention to use massage during childbirth.

MASSAGE KIT

For massage during childbirth, a popular choice of essential oil is lavender for its sedative effect and fresh aroma (*see* Choosing and Blending Oils, *pages 14–15*). The scent of oils in the room can be very soothing. Ask the doctor if you can use an oil burner or electric vaporizer: each device has a bowl that can be filled with a little water and 2–4 drops of essential oil.

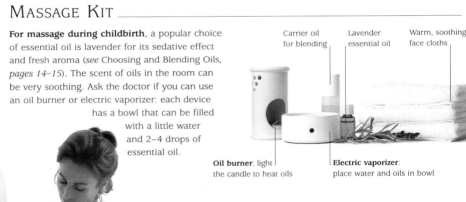

Carrier oil for blending

Lavender essential oil

Warm, soothing face cloths

Oil burner: light the candle to heat oils

Electric vaporizer: place water and oils in bowl

LOWER BACK & LEGS

1 For this sequence, ask your partner to lean forward, using the wall as a support. Kneel beside her and apply circular palm pressures all around the sacrum with your right hand, as your left hand supports the area. Then stroke the area gently.

2 To ease lower back pain, support the buttocks with your fingers and press deeply into the center of each buttock with your thumbs. Hold for a few seconds, then release.

3 ◄ Continue the massage by stroking softly down the backs of the legs with each hand. Your partner may want to shift her weight from one leg to the other.

4 As a further way to ease pain and speed up delivery, press on the shiatsu point on the inside of the leg four finger-widths above the ankle prominence in the groove behind the shinbone.

MASSAGE AFTER CHILDBIRTH

AFTER THE MENTAL, EMOTIONAL, AND PHYSICAL STRAIN of childbirth, new mothers need to be nurtured themselves, and massage is a perfect way to relax the mind and body, renew energy, encourage deep sleep, and help the body regain its shape. In non-Western cultures, it is common for an extended family member, usually the grandmother or an aunt, to massage the mother on a weekly or daily basis during her "lying-in period," about 30 to 40 days. Below are a few abdomen massage techniques that I learned from midwives in India and Sarawak. Only do abdomen massage after the mother's post-partum check-up, generally about six weeks after the birth.

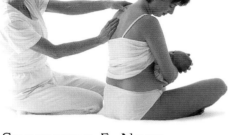

SHOULDERS & NECK

This area is often tense from breast-feeding, so loosen tight muscles with circular thumb pressures. Support a shoulder with one hand and work the thumb of your other hand all around the neck and shoulder blade, avoiding the spine. Repeat on the other shoulder.

ABDOMEN

1 ▶ Support the abdomen with your right hand and make a "V" shape between the thumb and fingers of your left hand. Stroke up from the pubic bone towards the navel with the "V", imagining that you are scooping everything back into place. Glide back and repeat three times.

2 Place one hand on top of the other and stroke very, very slowly and deeply up the abdomen. When you reach the navel, release the pressure and glide gently back. Repeat three times.

3 Gently circle around the abdomen, using soft and molding hands.

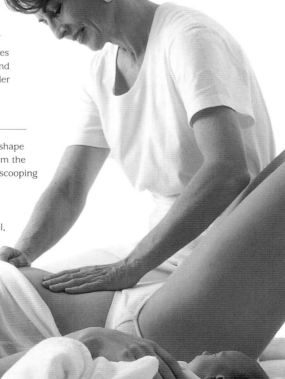

BABY MASSAGE

İT IS THE MOST NATURAL THING IN THE WORLD for new parents to stroke, cuddle, and rock their babies, and massage is no more than an extension of this desire to hold, touch, and provide comfort. Not only is massage a pleasurable, bonding experience for both parent and child, but it also encourages the baby to become responsive and sociable. Calm, soothing strokes help to ease anxiety and minimize crying, and research has shown that massage can boost a baby's immune system, lower stress levels, relieve colic, and encourage sleep. Although relatively new in the West, baby massage is commonplace in more traditional cultures, such as India and Africa.

> ❛ It is through our hands
> that we speak to the
> child … our hands that
> touch and hold. ❜
>
> FREDERICK LEBOYER,
> OBSTETRICIAN AND AUTHOR OF
> LOVING HANDS, 1976

PREPARATION

Babies feel the cold more than adults, so ensure that the room is warm throughout the massage. Make sure that you are both comfortable. You may want to massage your baby on the floor, in which case pad the area well with a futon or large, soft towels. Alternatively, sit up, leaning against cushions with your knees bent and your baby on your lap. Some babies like a rolled-up towel placed under their chests. The best time to massage is between feedings, after a bath, or simply when you both feel the need for closeness. The length of the massage depends entirely upon how long your baby enjoys it. I use a light, unscented oil (see page 14).

RESEARCH

Loving contact between mother and baby affects a child's development. In a 1992 study in London, England, levels of the stress hormone, cortisol, were seen to decrease consistently in premature babies after massage. In 1986, at the Miami Medical Center in Florida, premature babies were given three 15-minute massages a day over ten days. They averaged a 47 percent greater weight gain per day than the infants who were not massaged, and were more alert and active. The massaged babies were also in hospital for an average of six days less.

HEAD & FACE

1 Cup your baby's head with your hands. Hold for a few seconds, then very gently increase the pressure of your hands. Release, then, working from the centre outwards, make gentle circles to cover the whole head.

2 Support one side of the head with one hand and, with the thumb and fingertips of your other hand, gently squeeze and pull the ear. Swap hands to support the other side of the head, and work on the other ear.

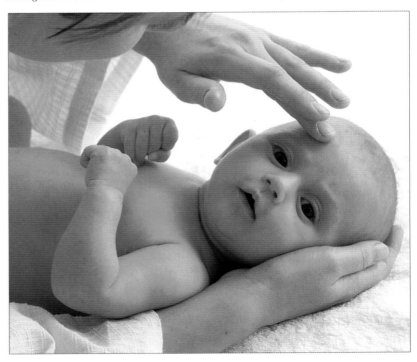

3 With one or both thumbs, stroke from the center of the forehead out to the hairline, then down to each ear. Stroke from the nose out to the ears, from the nose up to the forehead, and over the chin and jaw.

4 ▲ Now make soft, spiraling circles with your fingertips, circling the areas of your baby's face that you have just stroked. Finish by holding your baby's head in your hands again for a moment or two.

ARMS & HANDS

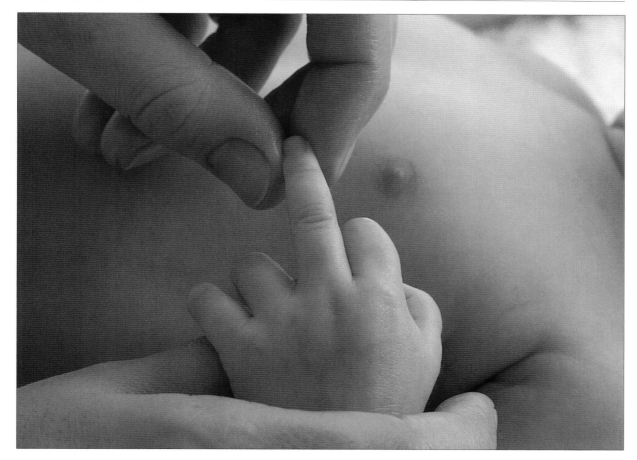

1 Pour some oil on your hands, place them on your baby's chest, and let the warmth gather. Stroke the left arm a few times, then gently roll it backward and forward between your hands.

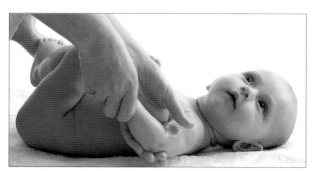

2 ▲ Rhythmically stroke one hand after the other down the left arm, then gently squeeze and twist the arm as you work down to the hand. Next, make soft circles around the elbow with one hand while the other hand supports the arm. Then stroke the hand itself, from the wrist to the fingers.

3 ▲ Play with each finger in turn, rotating and loosening the joints. Work between the knuckles and all over the palm, making bunny hop movements with your thumbs.

4 Now rub the left arm quite briskly, from the top to the bottom. This is a lovely energetic movement that can leave the baby gurgling with delight. Finish with soft feather stroking down the arm with your fingertips. Then move across to work on the right arm, repeating steps 1–4.

5 ▶ When both arms have been massaged, try some passive movements: stretch the arms in and out, across the chest, either one after the other or both of them at the same time.

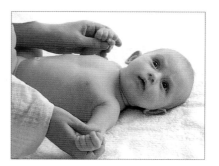

ABDOMEN

Stomach massage can help babies suffering from colic. By increasing the circulation and stimulating peristalsis, it can help to relieve gas and constipation. A good time to massage is when changing diapers, or before a feeding.

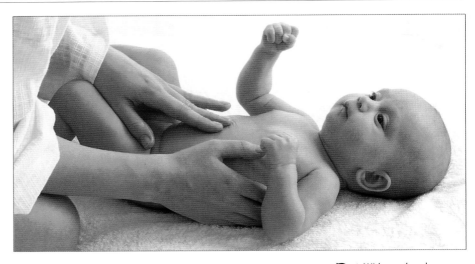

1 Hold both hands over your baby's stomach, then stroke one hand down and around in a clockwise direction, followed by your other hand (*see* Circle Stroking, *pages 26–27*). As one hand meets the other wrist, lift it over and complete the circle on the other side. One hand will therefore form complete circles while the other forms half circles.

2 ▲ With one hand as support, describe little circles all over the abdomen with the fingertips of the other hand. Start on the left side, and work in a clockwise direction around the area.

3 ▼ Bring your baby's knees up, over the stomach, and place the soles of the feet together. Relax your baby's abdomen by rotating the legs around in a clockwise motion. Try to keep the pelvis still as you circle the legs around. Then stretch the legs out, going backward and forward.

LEGS & FEET

Most babies love to have their legs and feet massaged. The strokes and movements encourage elasticity, flexibility, and coordination.

1 Stroke down the left leg from the hip to the foot. Then sandwich the leg with your hands and gently rock it up and down, and from side to side.

2 Gently squeeze and twist all the way down the leg to the toes, using either one or both of your hands. Then work up and down the leg with an energetic rubbing action.

3 Support the calf with one hand, and hold the ankle with your other hand. Slowly rotate the ankle, then move on to work on the foot.

4 ▶ Stroke from the ankle to the toes, then gently squeeze and rotate each toe. Repeat steps 1–4 on the right leg.

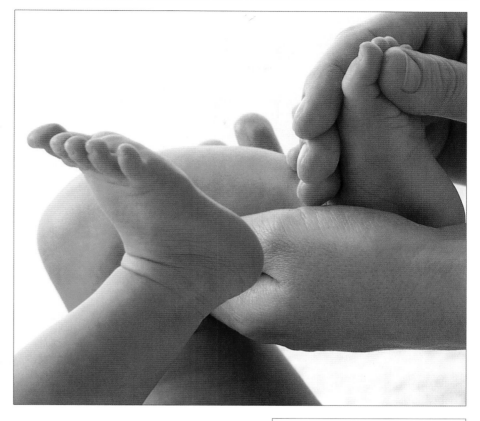

BACK

To massage the back, either lie your baby along your legs, or on the floor, or sit her up on your lap, leaning forward on to your arm.

1 Criss-cross, stroking across your baby's back. Use one hand if your baby is sitting, or both hands if she is lying down.

2 ▶ Stroke gently down your baby's back with the palm of your hand.

3 Make tiny circles with your fingertips, up and down the back on either side of the spine.

4 Finish by stroking your fingertips very lightly down your baby's entire back.

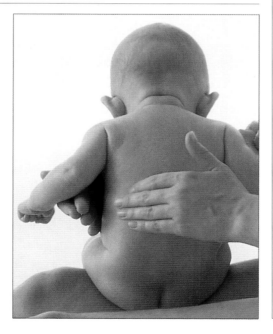

PRACTICE TIPS

Make sure that you are truly responsive to your baby during the massage. Start with your baby facing you, so that you can establish contact, and focus on the area to be massaged with your eyes before you introduce your hands.

◆

Begin by using the pads of your fingers to stroke slowly and gently. As both of you gain confidence, you can increase the rhythm and depth of the movements. You will soon learn your baby's likes and dislikes. Continue with the strokes as long as your baby is enjoying them.

◆

Your baby will react to your calmness and the confidence of your touch; the massage should be a pleasure for you both. The more relaxed you are, the more your baby will relax and enjoy the massage.

MASSAGE FOR CHILDREN

As CHILDREN GROW UP, there can come a time when physical contact with them is greatly diminished. Massaging your children, or asking them to massage you, is a wonderful way to stay in close contact. Children who no longer wish to be cuddled enjoy the formality of a massage, and a caring touch can encourage them to voice thoughts and concerns that may otherwise be difficult to express. Children are frequently shy and conservative, so it helps if you introduce massage in a way that will appeal to them. If they enjoy cycling or soccer, for example, offer them a leg massage; if they spend their lives reading, give them a face and shoulder massage. Then get them to give you a massage in return.

❝ The most sullen and morose child seems gradually to be imbued, under the influence of massage, with the attributes of a docile, willing and kindly disposition. ❞

DR. STRETCH-DOWSE,
LECTURES ON MASSAGE, 1895

RESEARCH

The following studies, carried out in the 1980s and 1990s, reveal the benefits of massage and touch on children.
A study at 16 primary schools in the Midlands of England by Birmingham University found that when teachers supplemented praise with a pat on the back, bad behavior was reduced and pupils worked about 20 percent harder.
In a US study by Touch Research International (TRI) in Miami, a 30-minute back massage was given daily for five days to 52 children and adolescents who were being treated for psychiatric problems. When compared to a control group who had viewed relaxing videos, the massaged patients were not only less anxious and agitated, but were also able to sleep better and were more cooperative. In another TRI study, one group of autistic children was given a massage twice a week for five weeks while another group played a game with a teacher who held each child for a similar length of time. By the end of the time period, the massaged children were reported to be calmer and more in control.

LEG MASSAGE

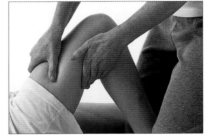

1 ▲ Begin by gently stroking your child's thigh. Ask him to bend his leg, then stroke one hand after the other firmly down the thigh toward his body. As each hand reaches the top of the thigh, return it to the starting position and repeat, trying to achieve a rhythmic effect.

2 Repeat step 1, but flex your fingers so that you create a deep, raking movement as you stroke down the thigh.

3 ▲ Try hacking the outer thigh: lightly strike the flesh with the sides of alternate hands, keeping your wrists loose and relaxed so that your fingers knock together. Finish this stage of the massage with gentle stroking.

4 ▶ Now continue on the calf with criss-crossing strokes. Mold your hands on the back of the lower calf, and pull them firmly toward you so that you squeeze the flesh. Push your hands gently back to the starting position and repeat. Work up the whole calf.

CHILDREN GIVING THE MASSAGE

Children can give a really good massage by the age of about five or six years, and the back is an easy place to start.

Ask your child to kneel behind you and to flex his fingers so that he can stroke down the back with deep, rake-like strokes. He can also try kneading your shoulders by squeezing and releasing them.

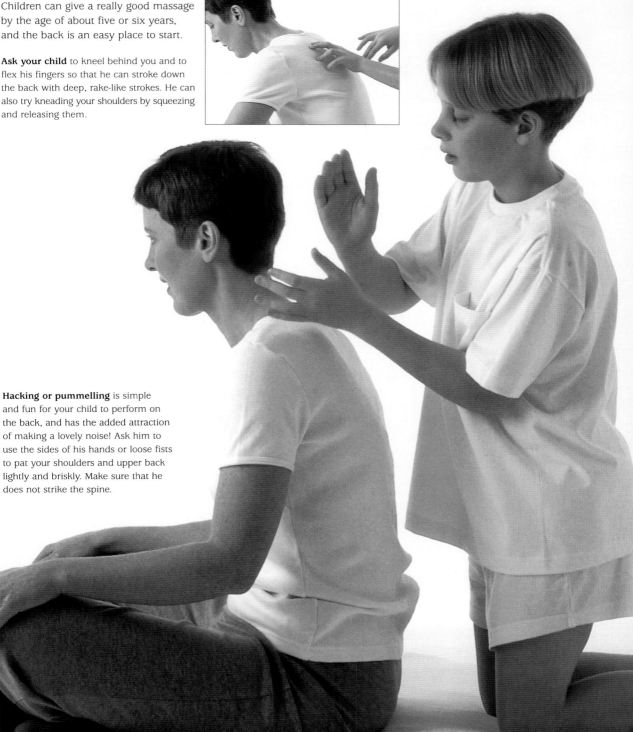

Hacking or pummelling is simple and fun for your child to perform on the back, and has the added attraction of making a lovely noise! Ask him to use the sides of his hands or loose fists to pat your shoulders and upper back lightly and briskly. Make sure that he does not strike the spine.

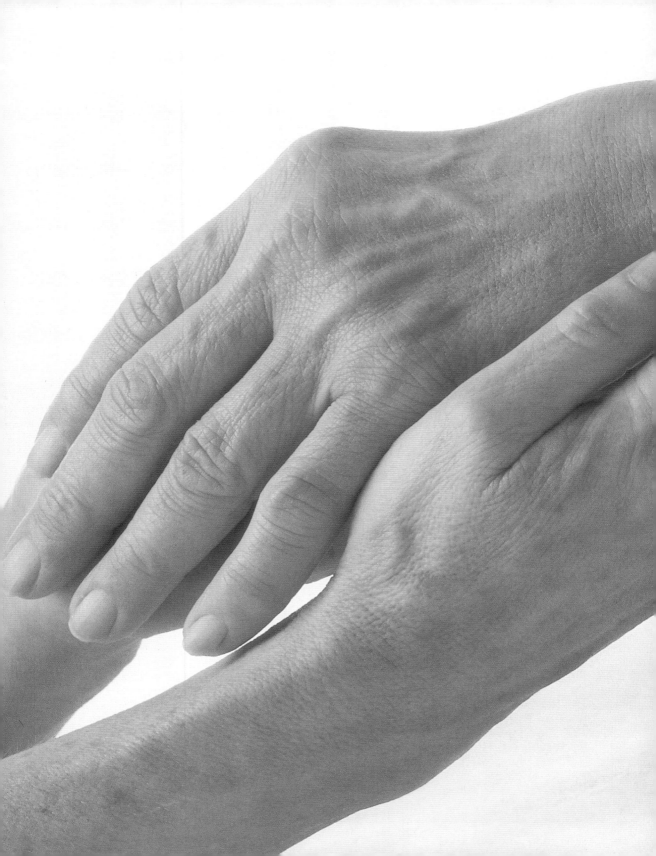

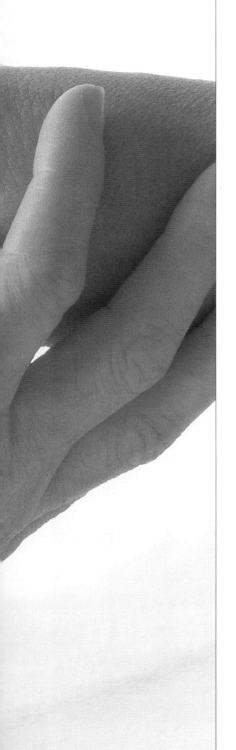

MASSAGE
FOR HEALTH

MASSAGE CAN PRODUCE A RANGE OF REAL PHYSICAL

AND PSYCHOLOGICAL BENEFITS. THESE CAN ENHANCE

FLEXIBILITY AND ATHLETIC PERFORMANCE IN A HEALTHY

BODY, OR CAN HELP A BODY THAT IS OUT OF BALANCE

OR STRUGGLING WITH SERIOUS ILLNESS. RECENT

MEDICAL RESEARCH STRONGLY SUGGESTS THAT

MASSAGE DECREASES SUFFERING IN ILLNESS,

REDUCING TENSION AND ANXIETY, AND PROMOTING

WELL-BEING, RELAXATION, AND CONTENTMENT.

MASSAGE FOR SPORTS

MASSAGE HAS A LONG HISTORY as an effective method of preventing sports injuries and enhancing athletes' performance. Galen (AD 130–200), for example, who was chief physician to the Roman Emperor Marcus Aurelius, recommended massage for the gladiators, both before and after exercise. Now, as then, top athletes follow this advice.

MASSAGE & EXERCISE

Regular massage is the perfect adjunct to exercise: it helps people who participate in activities as diverse as running, football, and ballet, to keep physically, mentally, and emotionally healthy. It improves their performance by keeping muscles at the peak of their flexibility and strength, and it reduces any unpleasant side-effects of heavy exercise, such as stiffness and muscle soreness. Sports massage also eases anxiety, keeping the athlete mentally alert, yet calm. People on a regular program of sports massage experience benefits such as improved speed, strength, and flexibility, and they recover from events more quickly than other athletes do.

SPORTS MASSAGE RESEARCH

A variety of studies has concluded that massage after strenuous exercise aids recuperation and reduces side-effects. In an American university research project in 1994, for example, 14 men performed arm exercises designed to produce muscle soreness. Two hours later, they either had a 30-minute massage or a rest. Results showed that massage helped to prevent the onset of muscle soreness.

Another study in 1995 compared the effects of massage and rest on people who had exercised vigorously. Compared to those who had only rested, those who were massaged between sets of exercise recovered more quickly and performed better in subsequent exercises. It is known that massage also helps to improve muscle strength. In a study in 1990 at the University of North Carolina, researchers checked the muscle strength of a group of men who were massaged after performing leg exercises. The massaged group's strength increased, while the muscle strength of the group who were not massaged decreased significantly. Also in 1989, in Aspen, Colorado, a group of researchers examined the effects of massage on muscle function. They concluded that massage increases muscular endurance and that it aids recuperation from fatigue more effectively than rest alone.

BENEFITS OF SPORTS MASSAGE

Relieves muscular tension.

✦

Softens and lengthens muscle fibres.

✦

Improves mobility and flexibility.

✦

Increases alertness and energy levels.

✦

Assists recovery and general well-being.

✦

Improves fluid exchange and circulation.

✦

Increases lymphatic drainage.

✦

Reduces scar adhesions in body tissue.

IMPROVING PERFORMANCE

Sports massage can be tailored to suit both pre- and post-event needs. A combination of sports massage and stretching exercises helps to prepare the body before an event, and to relieve muscular tension afterward.

If muscles are tense, they cannot perform to their maximum potential, and pre-event massage helps to prepare the athlete by relaxing the muscles in readiness for exercise. It also helps to reduce pre-event anxiety and to promote a calm, alert state.

❛ *Massage diminishes blood pressure but without increasing the activity of the heart; on the contrary, the heart's action is lessened in force and frequency. The contracting hands of the manipulator are, as it were, two more propelling hearts.* ❜

DR. GRAHAM, BOSTON, MA,
PRACTICAL TREATISE ON MASSAGE, 1902

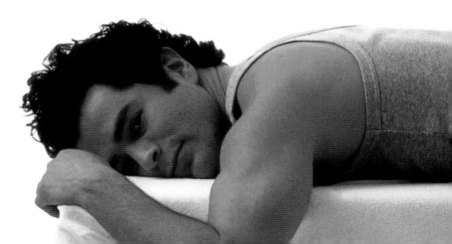

PRE-EVENT MASSAGE

Give a massage (as shown here) two to three days before the event, to help your partner feel relaxed and supple. A full-body massage is ideal but, if you are short of time, massage the main muscles your partner will be using, such as the legs. Athletes also benefit from massage an hour or so before an event, which should be light but stimulating, except if they are anxious, in which case try calming strokes (*see pages 20–31*).

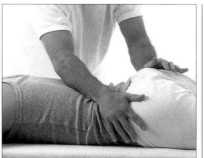

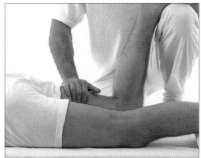

1 ▼ Begin with stroking, kneading, and rocking movements to prepare the area for deep tissue work. Use elbow pressure to soften tight muscles and promote mobility around the hip joint. Exert pressure in particular on the posterior muscles of the hip. Use the weight of your whole body for this deep compression technique, with one hand holding the ankle, and your other elbow and forearm carefully pressing into the gluteal muscles.

2 After deep tissue work, softer massage techniques help to restore blood flow to the area. Rhythmically grip and gently knead different sections of the gluteal muscles to soothe the area that you have been working on and to create a softening effect.

3 The hamstring muscle group benefits from being vigorously shaken to loosen it up. Place your leg on the couch and use it to support the leg being massaged. Use one hand to hold the foot and the other hand to pull the muscles slightly away from the bone, shaking the muscles rhythmically. This technique has a relaxing effect, both mentally and physically.

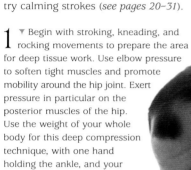

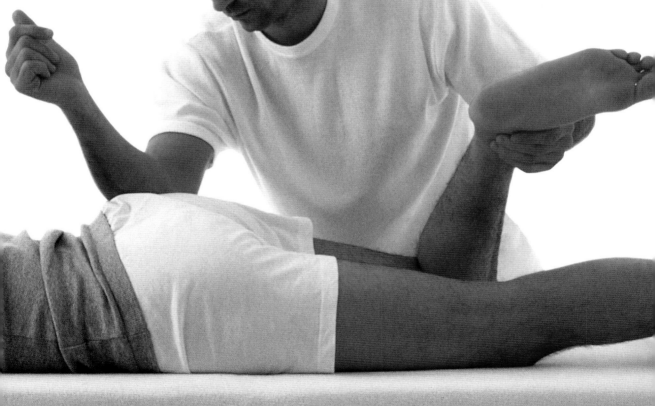

POST-EVENT MASSAGE

During exercise, waste products, such as carbonic and lactic acid, are produced by the muscles. In extended periods of intense sports training, the waste products build up, creating areas of deep muscular tension and stiffness that are the precursors of injury. Even the most comprehensive stretching program may not be sufficient to alleviate this tension, but sports massage can have a profoundly helpful effect because it softens and lengthens contorted muscle fibers and surrounding connective tissue.

PREVENTING STIFFNESS & INJURY

Massage after strenuous exercise helps to disperse accumulated waste products at a faster rate, particularly when it is combined with a regime of low-intensity cool-down exercises. Massage improves blood flow to the capillaries (tiny blood vessels) deep within the muscles, and it aids the circulation of lymph. Improved circulation within the muscles keeps them healthy because increased blood flow brings oxygen more efficiently to individual cells, and removes carbon dioxide. Improved lymph flow speeds up the rate at which waste products are removed from the muscles, helping to prevent stiffness.

Sports massage is also valuable for preventing the formation and build-up of fibrous (scar) tissue following an injury. During deep sports massage, any existing fibrous tissue can be stretched effectively by the therapist.

> *Its aim is double: to empty the exertions and to preserve the body from fatigue... But since the rubbing must be neither slow nor hard, we must pour oil plentifully over the body of the person who is rubbed; for this contributes to both the quickness and softness of the rubbing; and it enjoys also another very great advantage, for it relaxes tension and softens the parts that have suffered in the more violent kinds of exertion.*
>
> GALEN, AD 130–200

POST-EVENT MASSAGE ROUTINE

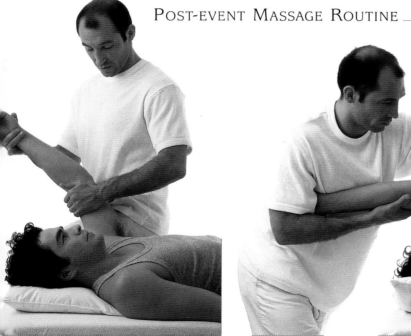

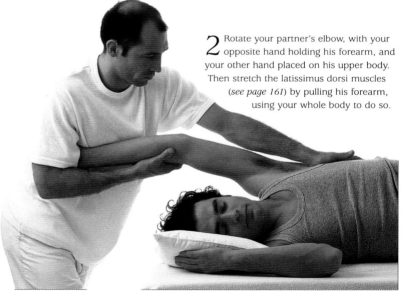

2 Rotate your partner's elbow, with your opposite hand holding his forearm, and your other hand placed on his upper body. Then stretch the latissimus dorsi muscles (*see page 161*) by pulling his forearm, using your whole body to do so.

1 Support your partner's arm with your hand to enhance lymphatic drainage. Squeeze the arm muscles with your free hand, as firmly as is comfortable for your partner. *Effleurage* (*see pages 64–65*) can also be performed from this position. Finish this stage by holding the hand and shaking the whole arm.

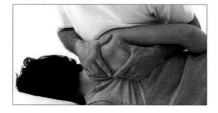

3 To stretch the rhomboid muscles (*see page 161*), ask your partner to roll on to his side. Next, place one hand under your partner's arm and the other over his shoulder. Tuck your fingers into his shoulder blade and stretch the muscle up towards you, while rocking the shoulder gently forward and backward.

POST-EVENT MASSAGE TECHNIQUES

The best techniques to use in post-event massage are those that encourage blood and lymph to drain toward the body core. Use light pressure at first, slowly increasing pressure, but staying within your partner's "comfort zone".

Squeezing a limb correctly is similiar to squeezing a sponge to extract water. As you squeeze, you encourage the circulation so that waste products from the muscles are flushed into the lymph system, and oxygenated blood is shunted into the muscle.

SELF-HELP MASSAGE TIPS

An effective technique you can perform on yourself is to push on a tight muscle to "trick" it into releasing. Do this by pressing the hands together on either side of the muscle; use the heel of the hand and extended fingers or fingertips. Do not slide, but pull or push the tissue together. Hold for a minute and very slowly release. This is very effective when used on the neck, and the trapezius muscle in the shoulders.

Cramp is caused by excessive muscular contraction (*see page 142*). You can relieve the pain by stroking and kneading the calf muscles and soles of the feet. This is particularly effective when combined with stretching exercises. If you are prone to cramp, you may find that soft-tissue massage and stretching before an event help to prevent it.

SPORTS MASSAGE CAUTIONS

If your partner has excessive swelling, increased temperature, or pain, treat them with basic first aid and seek medical assistance urgently. If your partner finds that muscle soreness makes them feel too tender to receive a sports massage, try MLD (*see pages 74–77*), which is also extremely effective and which is very gentle.

HELPFUL TREATMENTS

+ *Deep stroking* (see pages 32–33).
+ *Kneading* (see pages 34–37).
+ *Pressures and cross-fiber work* (see pages 38–39).
+ *Percussion movements* (see pages 40–43).
+ *Shaking and rhythmic movements* (see pages 44–45).
+ *Effleurage* (see pages 64–65).
+ *MLD* (see pages 74–77).

SELF-HELP

Self-massage complements stretching before the event; use direct pressure on trigger points and on any tight areas. Post-event massage combats muscle stiffness and fatigue.

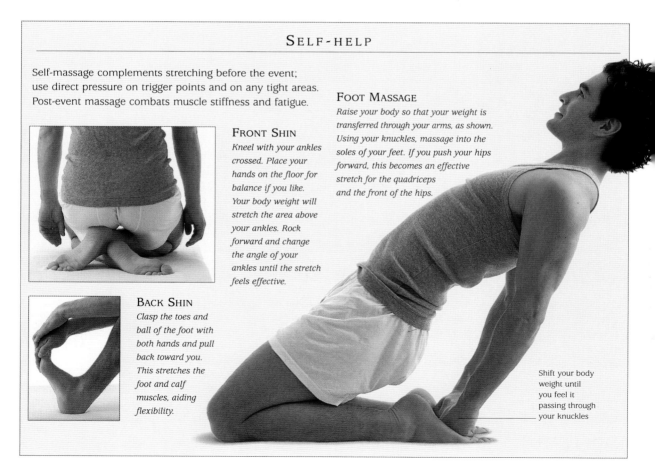

FRONT SHIN
Kneel with your ankles crossed. Place your hands on the floor for balance if you like. Your body weight will stretch the area above your ankles. Rock forward and change the angle of your ankles until the stretch feels effective.

BACK SHIN
Clasp the toes and ball of the foot with both hands and pull back toward you. This stretches the foot and calf muscles, aiding flexibility.

FOOT MASSAGE
Raise your body so that your weight is transferred through your arms, as shown. Using your knuckles, massage into the soles of your feet. If you push your hips forward, this becomes an effective stretch for the quadriceps and the front of the hips.

Shift your body weight until you feel it passing through your knuckles

REPETITIVE STRAIN INJURY

REPETITIVE STRAIN INJURY (RSI) has achieved notoriety in the workplace. It causes pain in the forearm, wrist, and hand, and is an occupational hazard for a variety of workers, ranging from machine operators and typists to massage therapists, who all repeat single movements over and over again. Massage can help to relieve the muscle tension that causes the pain.

A susceptibility to RSI can be inherent in a job itself, for example in road drilling, or it can be caused by the way a task is performed, for instance by sitting awkwardly when typing. Previous accidents or sports injuries can also make people susceptible to RSI, because the injuries create a muscle imbalance or joint problem that is then aggravated by undertaking repetitive tasks. RSI may also affect those who continually perform a task from the same side, rather than alternating when possible.

By dispersing muscle tension, both regular exercise and relaxation techniques can help RSI. It is also important to adjust equipment and furniture so that you do not have to twist your neck or hunch your shoulders while working.

Various massage techniques can help RSI. Kneading the shoulders and the trapezius muscle in the upper back, which supports the neck and head, reduces tension in those areas. Deep compression of the forearm muscles can also be very beneficial.

SELF-HELP

Take regular breaks from repetitive tasks.

✦

Try swimming, running, walking, and stretching. Regular exercise helps to prevent the build-up of muscle tension.

✦

To relax the body, lie on the floor with your knees up, and your head resting on a book. Contract and then relax the different parts of your body in turn.

HELPFUL TREATMENTS

✦ *Deep kneading (see pages 34–37).*
✦ *Pressures (see pages 38–39).*
✦ *Self-massage on the hands and forearms (see pages 60–61).*

CRAMP

CRAMP IS A SUDDEN, INVOLUNTARY CONTRACTION of a muscle, making it become taut and painful. It most commonly affects the muscles in the calves and feet, and can be agonizing. Massage, in the form of deep stroking and kneading, is excellent for cramp, helping to reduce tension, lengthen contracted muscle fibers, and relieve pain.

Muscles contract when they are being used to create movement or to hold a strong position. The latter creates more tension in the muscle than the former. If you hold a position when the joint is at the end range of its movement, for example if you extend your leg and point your toes, your muscles eventually will not be able to shorten any further and will go into a static reflex spasm (cramp).

Cramp can occur as a result of exercise, but the cause is not always known. It may sometimes be due to low levels of glucose, sodium, or calcium in the blood,

or due to dehydration. People with sedentary lifestyles, former ballet dancers, and those whose muscles have become chronically shortened, may be predisposed to cramp.

Deep stroking or kneading of the calves and soles of the feet can reduce tension, especially if combined with stretching.

HELPFUL TREATMENTS

✦ *Deep kneading (see pages 34–37).*
✦ *Leg and foot massage (see pages 56–57).*

SELF-HELP

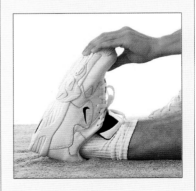

Stretch the foot for instant relief. Also try the sports massage stretches (see page 141).

✦

Exercise for at least 20 minutes three times a week.

ACHING FEET

I T IS ESTIMATED THAT THE AVERAGE PERSON walks about a thousand miles in a year, so it is not surprising that we sometimes have aching feet. Considering their importance, we give our feet very little care or attention, but regular foot massage can be most beneficial, helping to relieve the aches and pains that result from over-exertion and from standing for long periods.

A marvel of engineering, the foot is composed of 26 bones and an intricate network of muscles. The bones are arranged in a series of arches, which enable the foot to support the weight of the body and provide the leverage needed for walking. Any injury to the foot can disrupt the whole body, throwing out the musculo-skeletal alignment, which can cause problems such as backache and headaches.

We often treat our feet badly, forcing them into ill-fitting shoes, and we are usually only aware of them when they begin to ache. Prevention is the key to dealing with aching feet: choose comfortable, well-fitting shoes, and remove corns and calluses as they

occur. To strengthen the muscles of the feet, try to take the stairs rather than the elevator, and walk as much as possible, especially up hills.

The foot, particularly the sole, contains thousands of nerve endings, and massaging your feet regularly will not only relieve aching feet but can also revitalize the whole body (*see* Reflexology, *pages 98–99*).

> ❛ *The foot is probably the most*
> *neglected part of the body*
> *although it receives the greatest*
> *trauma of all.* ❜
>
> DR. ALBERT KLIGMAN,
> UNIVERSITY OF PENNSYLVANIA

SELF-HELP

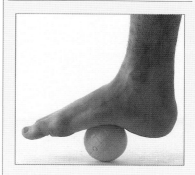

Roll your foot on a ball to exercise it, or try picking up pencils with your toes.

◆

Soak your feet in warm water, to which a few drops of lavender or rosemary oil have been added. Afterwards, rub away dead skin with a pumice stone.

◆

Massage your feet regularly (see pages 56–57).

SPRAINS & STRAINS

A SPRAIN IS CAUSED BY THE ABNORMAL WRENCHING and twisting of a joint. The ligaments, which hold the bone ends together, are stretched and torn, and the surrounding muscles, tendons, blood vessels, and nerves may also be damaged. A strain is a torn or stretched muscle. Gentle massage can help to ease both of these injuries.

At the first opportunity, place a cold compress, such as an ice pack or a package of frozen peas, on the injured area to reduce inflammation.

If the area is very painful or swollen, consult a doctor to rule out the possibility of fracture or dislocation. If massage is deemed an appropriate treatment by your doctor, try stroking

movements above the swollen area. These actions help to drain away the fluid and blood surrounding an injury that are the main causes of swelling. Sprains and strains can cause anything from mild discomfort to severe pain, so if you are massaging someone else, always ask them to tell you if the pressure is uncomfortable.

The muscles around an injury may become tense from the change in the way they are used, for example through limping. General massage of the surrounding area can dissipate the tension and pain that this causes.

SELF-HELP

Apply a cold compress for at least 10 minutes.

◆

Compress the area with a bandage and keep it raised.

◆

Try MLD (see pages 74–77).

STRESS

UNFORTUNATELY, AT SOME TIME IN OUR LIVES, most of us will experience some of the symptoms of stress. In fact it is estimated that up to a third of all sick leave is related to the effects of stress, anxiety, and depression. I have been helping clients cope with stress for 30 years, and I believe that massage has an important role in stress management.

"FIGHT OR FLIGHT" RESPONSE

When the body responds to a stressful situation, stress hormones flood the body, the muscles tense, the breathing rate increases, and the heart pumps faster. This reaction, which prepares the body for intense physical activity, is a legacy from our ancestors' "fight or flight" response. It would have helped them when faced with a threat, such as a predatory wild animal, to fight or to run away.

HARMFUL EFFECTS OF STRESS

We all need a certain amount of stress to give our lives zest and excitement. Stress only becomes a negative influence when the demands made upon us seem too great and we feel unable to cope.

The stress response anticipates physical action. But many stressful situations, such as worrying about how to pay a household bill, do not necessitate an immediate physical response.

Without intense activity to dispel stress hormones, our bodies suffer, giving rise to problems, such as irritability, fatigue, insomnia, depression, backache, headaches, anxiety, indigestion, and high blood pressure. Stress has a cumulative effect and in the long-term, it can contribute to an increased perception of pain, susceptibility to colds, and heart disease.

MASSAGE & MOOD

There is increasing evidence to show that mental and physical health are inseparable, and that, by relaxing the body, massage calms the mind. Massage relieves the strain of being constantly alert, inducing a feeling of well-being. My clients tell me that after a massage they feel more optimistic, tranquil, and full of vitality. The sheer pleasure of massage is good for us; it may even have a protective factor, helping to "inoculate" us against disease, according to Dr. D.M. Warburton, Director of Psychopharmacology at Reading University, England, who says that "pleasurable events have a protective effect that lasts for days." Researchers in the US, measuring immune function, have found that people who are in a positive mood are healthier than those who are not feeling optimistic.

Massage gives body and mind a "breathing space;" time to relax and let go. Escaping from our worries results in improved sleeping patterns and a more balanced outlook on life, which in turn helps us to cope with our problems.

ANXIETY & DEPRESSION

There is significant evidence that massage can alleviate anxiety. In 1982, researchers at Michigan State University, measured the stress responses of 32 nursing students after ten minutes of rest, after three and six minutes of slow, stroking back massage, and after another ten minutes of rest. The students' anxiety levels were tested every three

RELEASING STRESS

Use the thumbs and fingers of both hands to knead away tension in the shoulders and neck. Finish with slow strokes to induce relaxation.

minutes during the period, and results showed that six minutes of massage lowered autonomic arousal (*see page 161*), producing a relaxed state.

Massage can decrease anxiety even more effectively than most forms of exercise. In 1988, researchers at North Texas State University, compared the relaxing effects of different sports with 30 minutes of massage. They found that only jogging equaled massage at relieving tension and anxiety.

Massage also helps people to fight depression. Many people would agree with one of my students who wrote, "Massage strengthened my confidence and offered me the support I needed. It felt wonderful to be touched, cared for, and to feel valued. It led me to take an active interest in myself again".

LASTING EFFECTS OF MASSAGE

Massage makes it easier for us to cope with difficult situations and to recover from them faster. In 1990, at the University of North Carolina, volunteers were given mental arithmetic tests and a personal questionnaire. The following day, the subjects had either an hour of Swedish massage, or they relaxed and read a magazine. Afterward, both groups took the tests again, and it was noted that the massaged group was significantly less stressed during the tasks and recovered more rapidly than the other group.

My clients have been confirming this for years: they say that massage helps them through difficult periods of their lives, whether the difficulties be due to pressure at work or at home.

SELF-HELP

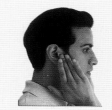

Try self-massage (see pages 48–61).

✦

Cut down on or give up cigarettes, alcohol, and caffeinated drinks.

✦

Exercise three to four times a week and eat a nutritious diet.

✦

Add a few drops of essential oils to a bath.

INSOMNIA

ALMOST EVERYONE SUFFERS FROM AN OCCASIONAL SLEEPLESS NIGHT but, for many, insomnia is a real problem. I find that one of the most satisfying aspects of massage is its ability to send someone to sleep. Soothing, hypnotic strokes can almost instantly induce a sense of calm that later can result in deep sleep.

RESTORATIVE SLEEP

About one-third of adults report chronic sleep problems and find that their sleeplessness leads to irritability, depression, impaired memory, and lethargy. People deprived of sleep are more susceptible to illness than usual, and both their productivity at work and their family lives can suffer.

As anyone who has had a massage knows, it is a profoundly relaxing experience. Dr. D.M.O. Graham writing in 1913 in Boston, MA, summed up the calming effects of massage as, "Upon the nervous system as a whole massage exerts a peculiarly delightful and at the same time profoundly sedative and tonic effect... For hours afterward the subjects are in a blissful state of repose,

they feel as if they were having a long rest, or as if they have returned from a long vacation."

I find that clients often fall asleep during a massage session and later report having had the best night's sleep ever. Massage seems to have a cumulative effect so, if you do not fall asleep the first time, persevere. With luck, the next time you have a massage the soothing strokes will work their magic.

RESEARCH INTO CHILDREN

In a study at Touch Research International, in Miami, FL, babies were either rocked or massaged. The babies who were rocked subsequently woke up when they were put down to sleep. But those who were massaged fell asleep

quickly when they were put to bed. Massage does not just help babies; in a US study, reported in 1992, adolescents in a psychiatric hospital either had a daily massage or could watch a relaxing video. The sleep of the massaged group improved significantly.

HEALING AROMATHERAPY

If you associate an essential oil with a relaxing experience such as a massage or a warm bath, in time you will find that scent soporific. In aromatherapy, chamomile, lavender, and sandalwood are all used for their sedative effect. Many who use them report that the oils help to break the cycle of insomnia, ensuring a good night's sleep.

HELPFUL TREATMENTS

✦ *Soothing cat strokes (see page 21).*
✦ *Face massage (see pages 51–53).*
✦ *Foot massage (see pages 56–57).*
✦ *Shiatsu (see pages 94–97).*

HEADACHES

IT IS A NATURAL REACTION TO RUB YOUR TEMPLES and forehead to soothe away a headache. There are numerous types of headache but a tension headache is the most common. This is often caused by fatigue and stress, which produce muscular tautness. Massage helps release this tension and has a generally relaxing effect, often lifting a headache almost magically.

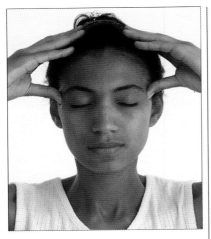

FACE MASSAGE
One of the fastest ways of lifting a headache is through face massage. To quickly diminish even the worst of headaches, first massage the back of the neck and head, then concentrate on the forehead, around the eyes, and on the temples. Very gentle, light stroking on the forehead also helps relieve even the most stubborn headache.

WHAT CAUSES A HEADACHE?
The muscular tension that causes most headaches occurs when muscles in the back of the neck and scalp contract. The blood vessels become constricted, preventing removal of metabolic waste products. This leads to tenderness and pain in the back of the neck, which can then spread to the head, temples, and around the eyes.

Headaches are commonly triggered by stress and anxiety, as well as by poor posture, eye strain, fatigue, and changes in the weather. If you regularly have headaches, you should consult a doctor to help determine the cause.

NECK & SHOULDER MASSAGE
By relaxing tense muscles, massage helps to restore blood flow and to dispel pain. Migraine support groups recommend any treatment that relaxes you as beneficial, but it has been found that treatments that focus on relaxing the neck and shoulders are particularly helpful.

This advice is backed by research. In 1990, in a study at Knopio University, Finland, 21 women suffering from chronic tension headaches each received ten relaxing upper-back massages over a period of two and a half weeks. Researchers found that the women had significantly fewer headaches immediately after the massage period, and that the rate remained low for months afterward. These results suggest that vigorous soft-tissue massage can have a beneficial effect on chronic tension headaches lasting for up to six months.

RELAXING SHIATSU
Some people who suffer from severe headaches find shiatsu helpful. Time and time again, headache sufferers have told me that they can control pain by massaging acupressure points, particularly those found in the hands, wrists, ankles, and feet.

In 1976, at the University of Illinois Medical School, Dr. H. Kurtland conducted a two-year study in which 200 people who suffered from headaches were taught to use acupressure techniques to help alleviate their pain. They applied pressure to the *Tai Yang*, Gall bladder 7, Large Intestine 4, and Lung 7 points (*see pages 94–97*) for

15–30 seconds. The results showed that shiatsu was effective in relieving the pain of both migraine and tension headaches, and that it replaced the need for painkillers.

THE ROLE OF ESSENTIAL OILS
Lavender oil is a well-known headache remedy; at the onset of a headache, mix eight drops with 20ml carrier oil and massage the mixture into your temples. Other oils with fresh scents that help to relieve tension include rose, chamomile, peppermint, and eucalyptus.

The results of a highly controlled research study in 1994, at the University of Kiel, Germany, confirmed that peppermint and eucalyptus essential oils can benefit headache sufferers. In the study, 32 people had eucalyptus oil, or peppermint oil, or a mixture of the two, diluted in a carrier and applied to

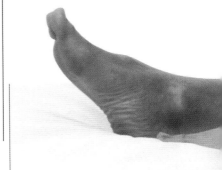

their foreheads. The results showed that peppermint and eucalyptus oils were relaxing, both physically and mentally, and that they increased cognitive performance. The study also found that peppermint oil mixed with eucalyptus oil had no effect on pain sensitivity. When used on its own, however, peppermint had a significant analgesic effect, and it reduced sensitivity to headaches.

❝ The head and hands should be rubbed gently to excite heat and in order that the strength of the body be increased. Later, let friction be performed on the head in an erect position and continued for some length of time. ❞

ARETAEUS, A FOLLOWER OF ASCLEPIADES IN ANCIENT ROME, ON RUBBING FOR HEADACHES, C.100 BC

HELPFUL TREATMENTS

- ✦ *Face massage* (see pages 50–53).
- ✦ *Neck and shoulder massage* (see pages 54–55).
- ✦ *Back massage* (see pages 68–69).
- ✦ *Shiatsu* (see pages 94–97).
- ✦ *Reflexology* (see pages 98–99).

SELF-HELP

Aromatherapy: apply essential oils, such as peppermint, to the temples (see pages 14–15).

✦

Massage your face, head, neck, and shoulders (see pages 50–55).

✦

Massage reflexology points on the toes (see pages 98–99).

✦

Apply a wet compress to the head.

✦

Try massaging your hands (see pages 60–61). Apply extra pressure around the base of the thumb and on the little finger.

✦

Shiatsu (see pages 94–97) can help. One of the best-known shiatsu points for headaches is the "Great Eliminator" (Large Intestine 4). This is situated between the thumb and the forefinger; press around the area until you find a point that usually feels quite distinctive. Do not press this point during pregnancy.

REDUCING TENSION

At the first sign of a headache, close your eyes and press between your eyebrows.

ABDOMINAL COMPLAINTS

DIGESTIVE PROBLEMS AND OTHER COMPLAINTS that affect the abdomen, such as premenstrual bloating, are common in developed countries. Poor diet and lack of exercise are some of the most usual causes, but emotional factors, including stress, also contribute to the problem. By alleviating pain and reducing stress, massage can help to relieve abdominal ailments.

BENEFITS OF MASSAGE

Releases muscular and emotional tension.

◆

Alleviates stress that exacerbates PMS and digestive disorders.

◆

Stimulates the movement of food through the gut.

ANCIENT SURVIVAL TACTIC

In response to stress, the digestive tract can react by producing excessive amounts of gastric acid and by causing the colon to contract strongly. It is not clear why this happens, but it may be a survival mechanism, dating back to when people depended on food from the wild. The severe colon contractions and the large amounts of gastric acid produced would have helped to protect the body from any poisons accidentally eaten. It may be that today our bodies still react to stress as if we have eaten a poisonous substance.

STRESS & THE DIGESTION

Stress is definitely a factor in digestive complaints such as constipation, diarrhea, and irritable bowel syndrome. Studies have shown that emotions such as excitement and anger affect the speed at which food passes through the intestines, sometimes with adverse results. In a survey in the early 1990s at the University of North Carolina, gastroenterologist Robert Sandler found that 49 percent of otherwise healthy people said that stress caused them abdominal pain, while 66 percent said that stress affected their bowel patterns, usually resulting in diarrhea.

REVERSING THE EFFECTS OF STRESS

A wonderful natural tranquillizer, massage is highly beneficial for anyone suffering from stress-related ailments, including premenstrual syndrome, and irritable bowel syndrome or other digestive problems. Massage soothes

pain, stimulates movement in the gut, and is calming, so helping to restore the working of the digestive tract to normal.

Stroking movements comfort and soothe body and mind, making the person feel cared for, which is immensely therapeutic as it reduces overall stress levels. I find that massage has a balancing, lightening effect on those who are tired, lethargic, and weighed down by stress. It also helps those who are hyperactive due to stress – they arrive feeling they cannot let go of their worries, and they leave feeling much calmer and more tranquil.

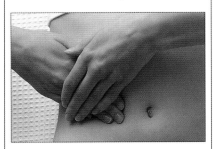

SELF-HELP FOR CONSTIPATION
Working in a clockwise direction, use your fingertips to apply gentle, undulating, circular pressures to the colon area.

CONSTIPATION & DIARRHEA

Massage helps constipation by relaxing the abdomen and by stimulating peristalsis (wave-like movements of the digestive tract that propel food through the system). In 1993, researchers at the Withington Hospital in Manchester, England, studied elderly patients with constipation. Instead of using enemas and laxatives, for 12 weeks the patients

exercised daily and had a ten-minute massage. Results showed that massage and exercise substantially reduced their need for enemas and laxatives.

Massage is not a new remedy for constipation – in fact medical books of the 19th century frequently advocated its use. One extreme suggestion of the time was to cure constipation by rolling a cannonball over the abdomen.

By helping to relieve stress, massage can alleviate diarrhea as well as constipation. Research at the University of Sheffield, England, on people with irritable bowel syndrome, found that stress played a strong part in the condition, but that it affected bowel function in different ways. In those prone to constipation, food moved more slowly through the colon when they were under stress whereas, in individuals prone to diarrhea, food moved more rapidly when they felt stressed. Massage can help relieve both ailments by reducing the stress that prevents the digestion from functioning normally.

PREMENSTRUAL SYNDROME

Symptoms of premenstrual syndrome (PMS) can vary from mild bloating and irritability to extreme aches and pains, and depression. Because massage is relaxing, it can soothe frayed nerves and generally induce a feeling of calm.

Many women have reported that some form of massage therapy was the most effective self-help method of relieving pain associated with PMS.

In addition, they said that massage, exercise, and relaxation alleviated PMS more successfully than any other treatment that they had tried.

If you suffer from PMS, as well as massage it is worth trying reflexology. In a reflexology trial in California, held in 1993, 35 women with PMS received eight half-hour treatments of either true or placebo reflexology. Those in the true reflexology group had both foot reflexology and stimulation of other reflex sites on the hands and ears. The points that were stimulated were those that correspond to the ovaries, uterus, pituitary glands, adrenal glands, and kidneys, and to shiatsu point Large Intestine 4 (*see* Shiatsu, *pages 94–97, and* Reflexology, *pages 98–99*).

Those receiving the placebo reflexology had treatment on sites not believed to be connected with PMS. The symptoms of those receiving true reflexology were reduced by 45 percent, compared to a reduction of 20 percent in the placebo group.

It is unclear whether these results are due to reflexology as we usually perceive it, or due to stimulation of accupressure points.

HELPFUL TREATMENTS

+ *Face massage* (see pages 51–53).
+ *Abdominal massage* (see page 58).
+ *Shiatsu* (see pages 94–97).
+ *Reflexology* (see pages 98–99).

6 *The effects of simple touch are quite remarkable. Pain is lessened… by the simple contact of the hand.* 9

DR. J. H. KELLOGG,
THE ART OF MASSAGE, 1895

POST-OPERATIVE RECOVERY

In a study at Kochi Medical School, Japan, in 1993, 16 patients who had undergone minor surgery under an epidural block were divided into two groups. One group acted as a control and the other group had a 30-minute stomach massage an hour and a half after the operation. The group who had received massage recovered faster from the epidural compared with the control group, implying that massage can help recovery after an operation.

SELF-HELP

Drink plenty of water and eat plenty of fresh fruit and vegetables to aid the passage of food through the intestines.

+

Take vigorous exercise, such as running, or swimming, three to four times a week.

+

Massage your stomach in a clockwise motion around the colon area. Also try applying undulating circular pressures (see page 58).

+

Try massaging the mouth and jaw (see pages 51–53). The gastro-intestinal tract is continuous from the mouth to the anus and massage around the mouth may help to ease digestive problems.

+

Press shiatsu points on the Stomach Meridian, such as Stomach 36 (see pages 94–97). Also, apply pressure to either side of the Achilles' tendon.

+

Try reflexology (see pages 98–99). For constipation, work on the colon, liver, and solar plexus areas of the foot. For PMS, work on the points on the outer ankle below the ankle bone.

RELEASING ABDOMINAL TENSION
Induce relaxation with calm, smooth stroking. Using both hands, gently stroke from the navel up toward the chest. Then let your hands glide out over the ribs. Ask your partner to tell you if the pressure is too strong.

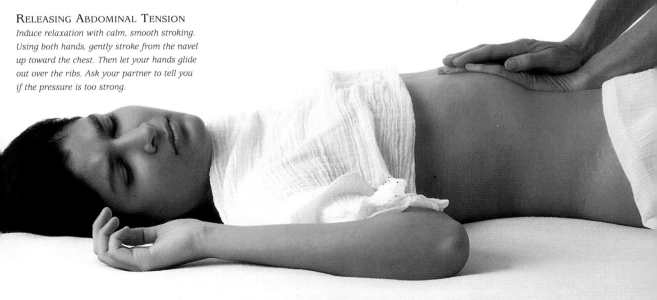

BACK PAIN

I T IS ESTIMATED THAT about 80 per cent of people in developed countries
have back pain at some point in their lives. The most usual cause is an
imbalance in the body. Whereas an ideal physique is balanced in terms of
flexibility and relative strength of left and right, most of us have backs that
are unbalanced in some way – strong but stiff, or flexible but weak.

COMMON CAUSES

A whole range of different factors
may contribute to back pain. Inherited
conditions or a previous injury, for
example, can create a predisposition
to backache. It can sometimes also
be linked to internal problems such
as constipation or gallstones.

   The most common cause of back
pain, however, is our lifestyle: sitting at
a computer for hours, driving, lack of
exercise, and ill-fitting or high-heeled
shoes make us vulnerable to backache.
Those involved in manual work, or in
sports that have a degree of assymetry
in them (tennis, for example), in the
long term may be prone to back pain.

TYPES OF BACK PAIN

Office workers, particularly those who do
not exercise, are prone to stiffness and
pain in the upper back. Excessive
stooping of the upper back is usually a
way of compensating for stiffness in the
lower back and legs, caused by sitting for
long periods. By contrast, those whose
work involves a considerable amount of
standing, lifting, or carrying tend to have
pain in the lower back. A bout of
excessive exercise or heavy gardening
can also cause lower back pain.

TREATING BACK PAIN

If you have long-standing or severe
back pain, you should be examined by
a professional, such as a doctor or an
osteopath, and you may need to adjust
your lifestyle.

   Once your doctor has confirmed that
massage is an appropriate treatment,
most styles of massage should help to
alleviate the pain. To relax taut muscles,

BENEFITS OF MASSAGE

*Relaxes stiff muscles that may be
contributing to back pain.*

Locates specific "trigger points" of tension.

Eases stress, often a factor in backache.

your back massage should include
compressing, broadening strokes, such
as deep stroking and kneading (*see pages
29 and 34–37*), which help to soften and
stretch the area, and restore the muscle
to optimum condition.

   If you are massaging someone with
back pain, you may come across points
that are particularly tender. These are
small areas of tension in the muscles
that are sometimes called "trigger
points." Deep, firm pressure or transverse
cross-fiber work (*see page 80*) can relieve
these points. Gradually apply pressure
and, as the area relaxes, slowly apply

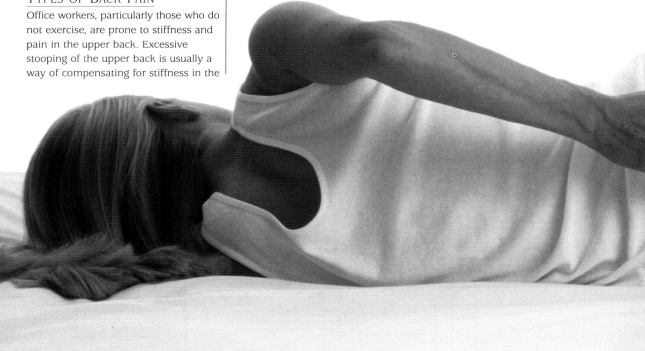

more pressure. If you feel the area beginning to tense up, decrease the pressure. After treating a trigger point, stroke and stretch the area to stimulate the circulation. Stress is connected to back pain (see Pain Research, below), so a relaxing massage will help you. See page 145 for other stress-management techniques. As well as massage, try lying flat on the floor; this is good for flattening the upper back. If you have lower back pain, you may need a pillow under your knees.

PAIN RESEARCH

Recent experiments at Pittsburgh University suggested that stressful thoughts lead to further pain in parts of the body that are already vulnerable. People were asked to describe their last episode of extreme pain and severe stress, while sensors measured their muscle tension. Those describing back pain showed a much higher level of tension in their back muscles compared with the control group or those describing other types of pain.

> 6 Upon the nervous system as
> a whole, massage exerts a
> peculiarly delightful and at the
> same time profoundly sedative
> and tonic effect. 9
>
> DR. D.M.O. GRAHAM, BOSTON, MA,
> PRACTICAL TREATISE ON MASSAGE, 1902

SELF-HELP

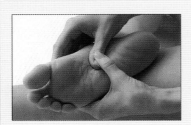

Massage the instep, which benefits the spinal area according to reflexologists (see pages 98–99).

✦

Lie down if you feel a stab of back pain, and apply a hot or cold compress to the area.

✦

Try gentle exercise such as walking or swimming.

✦

Learn to lift correctly: remember to bend your knees and keep your back straight.

✦

Check that your bed is firm.

HELPFUL TREATMENTS

✦ *Kneading* (see pages 34–36) of the legs, chest, abdomen, and the gluteal muscles in the bottom helps to relieve pain.

✦ *Skin rolling* (see page 37) and *Chinese massage* (see pages 78–81) disperse muscular tension in the small of the back.

✦ *Firm pressures* (see pages 38–39) can ease stiffness in a rounded upper back. Use them on the ribcage and upper back, in alternate directions.

✦ *Self-massage* of the neck, shoulders, and lower back (see pages 54–55 and 59) helps to relieve stress.

✦ *Back massage* (see pages 68–69) can ease pain. Use long, strong strokes down the back with the heels of the hands or the thumbs.

✦ *Thai massage* (see pages 86–89) is useful for stretching the back muscles.

✦ *Shiatsu*, (see pages 94–97). For upper back pain, including neck and shoulder pain, press the following points: GB20, GB21, LI10, Kidney 3, and Liver 3; to ease the pain of lower back pain, press these points: CV12, Kidney 3, and Liver 3.

✦ *Reflexology* (see pages 98–99).

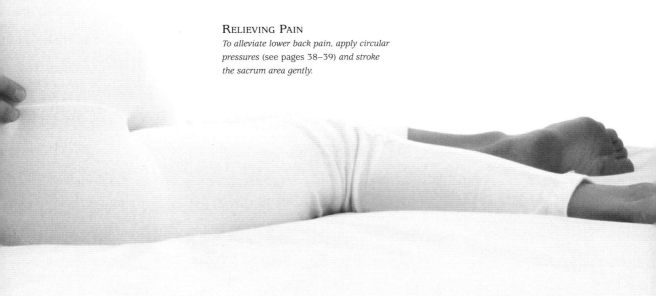

RELIEVING PAIN
To alleviate lower back pain, apply circular pressures (see pages 38–39) and stroke the sacrum area gently.

JOINT CONDITIONS

FEW PEOPLE GO THROUGH LIFE without experiencing some kind of problem with their joints. For example, osteoarthritis, which is one of the most common joint disorders, affects nearly 80 percent of those aged over 50. By relieving inflammation and improving flexibility, careful massage can be tremendously therapeutic for all types of joint condition.

OSTEOARTHRITIS

Also known as degenerative joint disease, osteoarthritis affects the hands, hips, knees, and spine. Usually, as a result of the ageing process, the cartilage lining the joints gradually degenerates, causing an affected joint to enlarge and become stiff and painful.

Gently massaging around painful joints can be very soothing because it improves the circulation. By stimulating lymph flow and the removal of waste products, massage helps to reduce inflammation and stiffness.

There are indications that dietary changes may also benefit people with osteoarthritis. Some nutritionists, for example, believe that cutting down on processed and acidic foods may help the condition. Relaxation techniques can also be useful, helping to relieve the muscle tension that accompanies stiff, painful joints.

In 1978, Stanford University, ran a six-week program for people with arthritis. Participants were taught about nutrition, how to overcome depression, and how to relax. After the program, those taking part reported that their pain had diminished by about 15 to 20 percent. They also said that they did not have to visit their doctors as frequently as before, and that their depression had eased considerably.

RHEUMATOID ARTHRITIS

Like osteoarthritis, rheumatoid arthritis results in swollen, painful, stiff joints. However, this type of arthritis has a very different cause – it is thought to be an auto-immune disorder, in which the immune system attacks the body's own tissues. While osteoarthritis is widespread among older people, those with rheumatoid

arthritis tend to be younger, with the disease most commonly affecting women aged 30 to 50.

Rheumatoid arthritis causes the synovial membrane, which lines the joints, to become thicker. The joints usually affected are the fingers, but the disease can also attack the knees, shoulders, and neck joints.

Massage above and below the swollen area has a two-fold benefit: by stimulating the circulation, it helps to decrease the inflammation and pain of swollen joints, and by soothing and relaxing the body, it induces a feeling of well-being that helps the sufferer to cope better with the disease. Research shows that feeling able to cope has a marked bearing on the condition. A recent study of 400 people with rheumatoid arthritis in the US, found that those with a strong sense of being in control of their symptoms experienced less pain and were in better health than those who felt defeated by the disease.

FIBROMYALGIA SYNDROME

Fibromyalgia Syndrome (FMS) affects about 2.5 percent of all women, but very few men. It results in widespread muscle pain and stiffness, and can include other symptoms such as irritable bowel, anxiety, depression, and headaches.

Massage can help FMS by reducing pain and stiffness, and by alleviating associated symptoms such as anxiety and depression. In a recent study at Touch Research International,

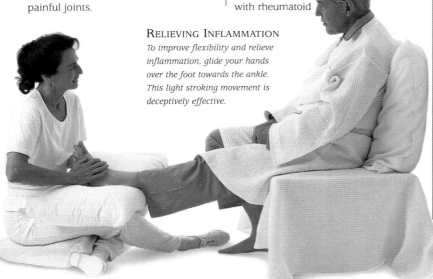

RELIEVING INFLAMMATION
To improve flexibility and relieve inflammation, glide your hands over the foot towards the ankle. This light stroking movement is deceptively effective.

Florida, FMS sufferers were massaged twice a week for five weeks. The levels of stress hormones in their blood were reduced after each massage, and they said that the massage course helped to reduce pain and stiffness, and to ease other symptoms such as insomnia.

MASSAGE FOR JOINT CONDITIONS

When you massage someone with a joint condition, avoid any area that feels hot and swollen: never massage directly on an inflamed joint. If a joint is only slightly inflamed, try massaging extremely gently above the site; this can be most soothing.

For arthritic joints in the hands that are not inflamed, stroke around the joint, then apply a very slight pressure to the joint itself with your thumb. Afterward, stroke the whole hand to soothe it. When massaging the hands, work around the wrist, the top of the hand, and the fingers, massaging toward the body to stimulate the flow of lymph.

The muscles around a damaged, arthritic joint sometimes react by going into spasm, which can cause intense pain. Massaging the whole area in a bath of warm water can be most comforting, helping to warm and soothe the afflicted part.

HELPFUL TREATMENTS

✦ *Gentle self-massage* (see pages 48–61).
✦ *MLD* (see pages 74–77) is a gentle and effective treatment.
✦ *Hydrotherapy* (see pages 120–121). Try soaking in a warm bath or applying hot and cold compresses to the area.

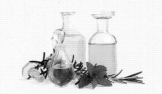
6 *Seized with rheumatic affliction of the left shoulder, I grasped firmly with my right hand about the middle of the pained muscle. To my surprise and huge gratification, I was instantly relieved from the pain.* 9

DR. BALFOUR, ILLUSTRATIONS OF THE POWER OF COMPRESSION IN THE CASE OF RHEUMATISM, 1816

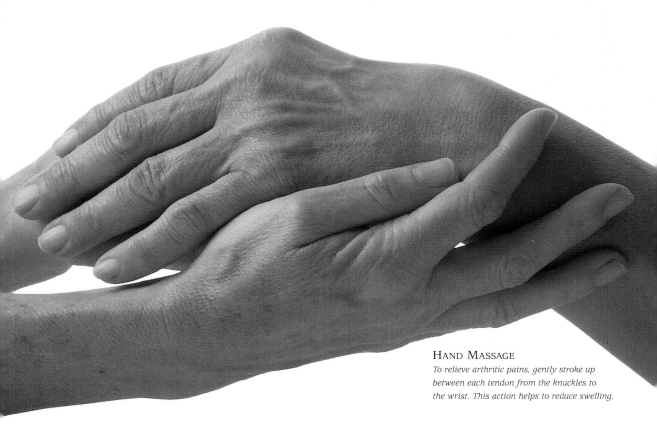

HAND MASSAGE

To relieve arthritic pains, gently stroke up between each tendon from the knuckles to the wrist. This action helps to reduce swelling.

MASSAGE & THE ELDERLY

IT IS NEVER TOO LATE to improve your health and quality of life. Massage can help you to achieve this goal by encouraging activity and vitality. Massage stimulates the circulation so that aches and pains are diminished, joints and muscles are loosened, and it is possible to become more mobile. Furthermore, the relaxing effects of massage induce a feeling of well-being and an optimistic outlook on life.

LIVING LONGER
In the developed world the fastest growing section of the population is the over-80s. As a result of improved diet and better standards of medical care, many elderly people remain active and busy, and continue to enjoy life. For others, however, the effects of ageing and inactivity mean that their lives are plagued by aches and pains, increased stiffness, less energy, and illness.

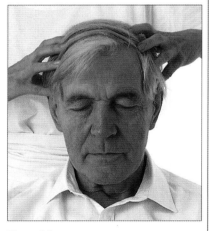

HEAD MASSSAGE
Gentle stroking massage of the head and scalp can be most soothing. It also communicates affection and empathy.

MASSAGE & FITNESS
Even people in their 90s can benefit from a fitness regime. The muscle strength of a group of 90-year-olds in Boston, MA, for example, increased by over 70 percent after an eight-week fitness course. Furthermore, the participants said they had found a new lease of life. Fitness in

old age is important because many of the changes we associate with ageing – decline in muscle strength, loss of bone density, aches and pains, joint stiffness, fatigue, obesity, and breathlessness – result from inactivity. Lack of movement also means that the circulation is impaired, waste products are not adequately removed, and the body is more prone to infection.

Stiff, painful joints can be major obstacles to participating in physical activity. By relieving muscular aches and pains, and loosening joints, massage enables elderly people to stay mobile and enjoy physical activities. As one of my clients said to me, "After my hand massage, I can do things for myself again. My hands are less puffy and stiff, and more supple."

In 1996, a study in the UK supported by the charity Age Concern found that massage can have a beneficial effect on mobility. Elderly people at various residential homes were massaged weekly. The majority of the participants experienced a reduction of muscular tension, particularly in their necks and limbs. The pain of immobility and arthritis was strikingly relieved in some cases.

LESS NEED FOR PAINKILLERS
Massage may offset the need for pain medication in elderly people, according to a US report by Touch Research International, Florida. Massage releases endorphins into the system, which are the body's own "feel-good" substances that raise mood and decrease perception of pain.

BENEFITS OF MASSAGE
Eases stiff aching joints, relieves pain, and increases flexibility.

◆

Improves the circulation.

◆

Communicates love, care, and concern.

◆

Relieves depression.

Helen Passant, a senior nurse at the Churchill Hospital, Oxford, England, uses aromatherapy as part of her care regime for the elderly. She finds that, as a result of regular massage, her patients need fewer prescribed drugs compared with patients on similar wards, and, in particular, they require fewer sedatives.

SKIN CARE
With age, the skin becomes thinner, losing its elasticity. Massage has a two-fold benefit: it increases the circulation, "feeding" the skin by bringing more nutrients to it in the bloodstream, and the oils used in massage soften the skin. Massage and essential oils can also help to heal ulcers and to relieve other skin conditions that may occur with age.

CARING TOUCH
The elderly often suffer from impaired hearing, sight, and mobility, which can make them feel vulnerable. For someone whose body is a source of pain or embarrassment to them, the caring non-judgmental touch of a massage is incredibly therapeutic. Touch can communicate love, care, affection, and empathy, and can make an elderly person feel comforted and serene.

In particular, touch seems to be very effective in reducing anxiety. In 1992, a study at Athabasca University, Alberta, Canada, discovered that a group of elderly people who received back massage while they were chatting to researchers were less anxious than another group of elderly people who had conversation-only sessions.

IMPROVING MENTAL CLARITY

Several studies have shown that touch can improve both attention and physical response in elderly, confused patients. For example, in 1982, in a simple experiment, patients were asked to complete a basic task. For some of the patients, the command was accompanied by a light touch on the forearm from a nurse. Compared with the others, those who were touched replied to the nurse more clearly and paid more attention to completing the task.

MASSAGING AN OLDER PERSON

In many respects, massaging an elderly person is no different from massaging anyone else, but you should bear a few points in mind. An older person's bones are not as strong as a younger person's, and they are more likely to have osteoarthritis. With age, the circulation tends to be less efficient, leading to cold, and sometimes painful, hands and feet. The skin becomes thinner as people get older, losing its elasticity, and it is more easily damaged.

When you massage an elderly person, remember that, as always, the receiver is in charge. Start gently and slowly, increasing the pressure to suit their preferences. It is easy to assume that, if someone is a little frail, they would automatically prefer a gentle massage. However, you may find that they like fairly firm pressure in certain areas, for example if they suffer from stiff shoulders. If the receiver finds it uncomfortable to lie on their stomach for a back or shoulder massage, they can sit at a table and lean forward on to pillows.

Try to pay particular attention to any areas of concern, and to the hands and feet. Massage will improve the circulation to the extremities, and will increase the flexibility and mobility of the joints. Massage the hands or feet with the receiver sitting in a chair. Support the arm or leg that you are massaging, so that the receiver can relax. Begin gently and slowly, only increasing the pressure if they wish. Be aware of thin skin or inflammation, (*see* Joint Conditions, *pages 152–153*), and moderate the pressure of your strokes to suit. Using gentle movements, rotate, flex, and extend the wrist and ankle joints to improve flexibility.

MUTUAL BENEFITS

The advantages of massage are two-fold, benefiting both the giver and receiver. It has been found that, in some circumstances, giving a massage can be even more beneficial than receiving one. In a recent experiment at Touch Research International, Florida, a group of volunteer "grandparents" massaged babies. Results showed that the elderly people derived more benefit from giving the massage than from receiving a massage themselves. They had fewer anxious and depressive symptoms than usual, made fewer visits to the doctor, and their self-esteem improved.

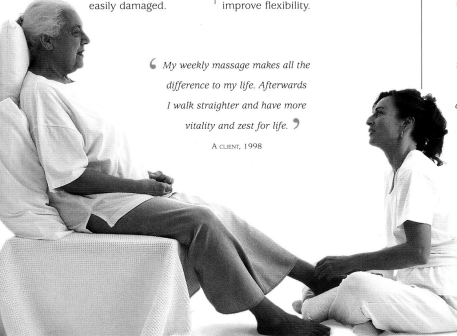

❝ My weekly massage makes all the
difference to my life. Afterwards
I walk straighter and have more
vitality and zest for life. ❞

A CLIENT, 1998

❝ If relaxation, touch, personal
warmth and a calming influence
have such profound effects... the
use of alternate therapies... should
be extended and made easily
available as part of the care system
in long-term situations. ❞

DR. JONES ON THE RESULTS OF THE
AGE CONCERN PROJECT, 1996

HELPFUL TREATMENTS

✦ *Foot massage* (see pages 56–57).
✦ *Hand massage* (see pages
60–61).
✦ *Shoulder and back massage*
(see pages 68–69).

MASSAGE & ILLNESS

WHEN WE BECOME ILL, we experience not only physical discomfort but also many psychological reactions. Whether we are suffering from pain, nausea, weakness, or fear, massage can help by conveying acceptance, support, care, and concern. I have worked with ill people for 30 years, and it still amazes me that something as simple as a massage can bring such benefits.

EXPRESSING CONCERN

If a friend is ill, it can be difficult to know how to respond, or what to say. Massaging an ill person is a practical way of showing that you care. Your concrete action expresses more than other forms of good wishes: it is one of the best and simplest ways of giving emotional support. When someone is ill, they may not want to talk, or they may not have the energy to do so. Through touch, however, you can reach out to them without the effort of conversation. Warmth, comfort, concern, and safety are all communicated through your hands.

THE VALUE OF SUPPORT

It is important to express our fears when we are ill. During or after a massage, I find that even the most reticent of clients will usually talk more freely, which, I think, is not only due to the relaxing effect of the massage, but also to the undiluted attention and support that they receive.

The value of support during illness was demonstrated in an American study in the 1970s by Dr. Spiegal. He found that women with breast cancer who participated in a support group lived on average for 18 months longer than those who received standard treatment but did not belong to a support group.

BODY & MIND CONNECTION

Recent research from the US reinforces the view that the health of the mind and the body are closely linked. According to the internationally renowned neuroscientist Dr. Candace Pert, old patterns of emotions are thought to be stored in nerve cells of the spinal cord and other parts of the nervous system. By activating these areas through touch, massage affects the mind. The action of massage induces a relaxation response and causes neuropeptides, which are chemical "messengers," to flow through the nervous system to the brain. The most well-known of the neuropeptides are endorphins, which generate pleasurable and optimistic feelings. Dr. Pert says, "When people feel pleasure they focus on the present moment rather than stay involved with worries or preoccupations."

Dr. Pert also suggests that anxiety, hostility, and other emotional states may have an adverse effect on the immune system, which is concerned with fighting infection. By lowering anxiety, improving mood, and inducing relaxation, massage has an important role in boosting the immune system and promoting good health.

HEART DISEASE

Early in my career, I worked on the cardiac ward at Charing Cross Hospital, London. Some of the patients had undergone heart surgery, others were recovering from heart attacks and they all suffered from high levels of anxiety.

One of the benefits of massage is the way that it can demonstrate what relaxation actually feels like. Before giving a massage, if I asked a patient to relax, they would often shout back tensely, "I *am* relaxed", but the gentle, soothing strokes soon induced a sense of calm. The patients could then compare their states of mind before and after the massage.

We found that massage helped patients to sleep and that it lowered their blood pressure and heart rate. These findings are backed by research. For example, a study in 1994 at the Middlesex Hospital, London, of 100 patients recovering from cardiac surgery, revealed that a 20-minute foot massage lowered anxiety rates, decreased pain, and reduced tension.

At Charing Cross Hospital, an important part of our rehabilitation program involved teaching couples how to massage each other so that the patients could continue to receive beneficial massages once they had returned home. If you are caring for someone with a heart condition, massage can be most helpful, although you must get their doctor's approval before you start. Try a gentle full-body massage with firmer strokes moving towards the heart and light strokes gliding away. If the person has had heart surgery, avoid the chest area until the scar has completely healed.

> ❝ With hope and expectancy comes remembered wellness, messages of healing that mobilize the body's resources and reactions. ❞
>
> HERBERT BENSON,
> TIMELESS HEALING, 1996

CANCER

Over the last 15 years, I have seen massage become widely accepted as a way to improve the physical and emotional well-being of cancer patients. In particular, it is effective in alleviating some of the unpleasant side-effects of cancer treatments, such as pain, nausea, and tension. In 1995, the Royal Marsden Hospital, London, conducted research in which 24 cancer patients had eight weekly massages with either plain or aromatic oil. Compared with a control group, the massaged group were less anxious, more relaxed, had less pain, and were more mobile.

It used to be feared that massage might actually spread cancer through the body, but there is no evidence for this. In fact Carl Simonton, the Medical Director of the Cancer Counselling and Research Centre, Dallas, TX, has been advocating massage for his patients since 1978. He states, "There is no contraindication to good therapeutic massage for people with cancer," and goes on to say, "Good therapeutic massage is massage done by a well-trained massage therapist, who is sensitive to the problems of massaging people with cancer, and is comfortable with people who are seriously ill."

There are no special techniques for massaging someone with cancer. However, as with all serious conditions, it is important to check with the person's doctor that it is an appropriate treatment. Any kind of touch is comforting; if your friend is confined to bed, a hand, foot, or face massage can be soothing. You may find that your friend has very dry skin, which is a side-effect of chemotherapy. If so, the massage oils will help to make the skin feel smoother and softer.

MASSAGE & AIDS

Acquired Immune-deficiency Syndrome (AIDS) is a condition in which the human immunodeficiency virus (HIV) invades and destroys cells that fight infection. Students from my massage school first worked with HIV-positive patients in the 1980s at the Mildmay Hospital in London. All the patients said how important massage was to them. It made a positive contribution to their lives: as well as diminishing physical discomfort, it made them feel cared for and supported.

Touch Research International in Florida in 1995 conducted a study on HIV-positive men to determine the effects of massage on the immune system. The participants received 45 minutes of massage five days a week for a month. At the end of the study, levels of the stress hormone cortisol had decreased, and levels of serotonin, a hormone that enhances mood, had increased. Even more significantly, the participants were producing more of the cells that fight invading viruses and bacteria.

ABUSE

People who become addicted to drugs or alcohol, or who have been sexually abused often suffer from poor self-esteem. Massage makes them feel special, so improving their self-respect. It can be an integral part of the healing process, putting people back in touch with their bodies, and helping the beginning of their recovery. Massage calms mood swings and panic attacks, and the relaxing, safe environment that massage takes place in can make a person feel accepted.

Many of my clients say that massage helped them to deal more calmly with difficult situations. As Ros Smith, who works for the British charity Turning Point says, "Massage acts as a safety net to anyone trying to put their life back on track… it can help change lives."

Drug addicts may have poor circulation and suffer from cold hands and feet. Massaging the extremities will improve their circulation, stimulate the release of neuropeptides and promote a feeling of well-being.

EMOTIONAL CONDITIONS

Massage can be of tremendous help for depression, for other types of mental illness, and for grief. It is something tangible that you can do for someone in distress. Often it is hard to find suitable words, but the hands communicate directly, offering comfort and empathy.

Some people, however, find that massage after a bereavement is initially too much for them; it releases too many of their emotions at a time when they are trying to keep themselves together. If this is the case, a little massage in time may help, once the initial pain has slightly subsided. You do not need to do a full-body massage to show that you care. Stroking the person's hands or massaging their shoulders can be most comforting.

UNIVERSAL BENEFITS

The examples of research given on these pages, plus the many more that exist, all indicate the enormous benefits of massage for those who are ill. Massage should be an integral part of caring for anyone who is sick in body, mind, or spirit. It provides tender loving care and soothes away pain and anxiety. Indeed, I believe that massage should be included as a part of every health care program, irrespective of the disease, in order to improve the quality of life. As Dr. Pert once said, "I almost cannot think of any aspect of medicine where the application of massage therapy would not apply."

HELPFUL TREATMENTS

+ *Aromatherapy* (see pages 14–15). Try soothing oils, such as chamomile or lavender, if discomfort is interfering with sleep. Uplifting oils, such as clary sage and geranium, can help lift depression.
+ *Self-massage* (see pages 48–61).
+ *Hand massage* (see pages 60–61) is useful if someone is confined to bed.
+ *Swedish full-body massage* (see pages 64–69) can help to ease pain.
+ *MLD* (see pages 74–77) is beneficial for congestion, helping to clear blocked sinuses or headaches, for example.
+ *Shiatsu* (see pages 94–97) is good for controlling pain and nausea.

MASSAGE IN HOSPITAL

STAYING IN HOSPITAL CAN BE EXTREMELY STRESSFUL. Patients have to contend with a strange environment, separation from loved ones, pain, anxiety about impending operations, and difficulty in sleeping. Massage is increasingly being used in hospitals to help people cope with these problems and to aid their recovery.

HEALING TOUCH

When you are in hospital, you become acutely aware of the way that people touch you. The difference between expressive, caring touch and procedural touch is huge. One patient I know summed it up as, "In hospital I was poked and prodded but never *touched*." Fortunately, this impersonal type of care is less common as more nurses become aware that touching and soothing are integral to good nursing. Massage is now being used in a variety of situations, including pediatric, psychiatric, and intensive care wards, and day centers and hospices. It can be incredibly therapeutic: one patient described the effect of massage to me, "The massage helped me not only physically but mentally. It was the catalyst to my recovery."

Massaging people in hospital has a further benefit. Both nurses and friends and relatives of the patient find it helpful to be able to provide comfort for the ill person. To quote one of my students at the Royal College of Nursing in London, "Massage fulfils a need for both the nurse and the patient."

REDUCING ANXIETY

Massage can be extremely useful in reducing anxiety because it helps to slow down the heart rate and relieve stress. A study held in 1974 in the US shows that human contact has a dramatic effect on heart response. In the study, the heart rate of patients in coronary care decreased by 20–30 beats per minute when a nurse touched and comforted them; an effect that was observed even when patients were in a coma.

Whether on the wards, or in out-patient departments, massage has a wide range of applications. Nurses find that it helps patients who are prone to panic attacks, for example, and that it is a good way of relaxing needle-phobic patients before an injection. It is not always necessary to give a full-body massage for the results to take effect. Even a ten-minute massage given to patients waiting for chemotherapy can help to reduce anxiety, making the treatment less traumatic.

PAIN & INSOMNIA

As well as relieving anxiety, massage can help to soothe pain. In 1988, at St. Mary's Hospital in London, 30 surgical patients had their faces, backs, and feet massaged. Afterward, researchers monitored them for physiological changes. They found that, compared with a group who had not been massaged, most of the massaged group reported less pain, less muscle spasm, and less anxiety. The patients who had been massaged also slept more soundly and reported improved well-being. There was a further benefit: the two nurses who performed the massage found that their rapport with the patients had improved as a result.

Pain can often cause insomnia and, at a number of hospitals, massage and aromatherapy are now being used to help patients sleep. When I work in hospitals, I often find that patients fall asleep after just a few minutes of massage, and time and time again, nurses whom I have trained tell me that they use massage to help anxious, sleepless patients drift off. Staffs report that the quality of patients' sleep improves dramatically as a result of massage and aromatherapy.

AIDING THE HEALING PROCESS

A recent American study, conducted by Professor Janice Kiecolt-Glazer at the Ohio State University, OH, suggests that stress impairs the body's ability to heal. Researchers monitored 26 women with identical flesh wounds to see how well they healed. Half of the volunteers were under considerable stress because they were caring for relatives with dementia. After the first five weeks, the wounds of nearly half of the control group had healed, compared to only 15 percent of the stressed caregivers.

I think this has important implications for people undergoing surgery. I believe that, since massage is known to reduce stress levels, massage before and after an operation will speed healing.

Research has shown that massage reduces both pre- and post-operative pain and anxiety, thereby helping the healing process. In 1993, for example, an Australian study compared the anxiety levels of 60 patients undergoing surgery. Half of the group was given a 45-minute massage before their operations, and they were found to be much less anxious than the patients who did not receive a massage. A recent French study of 116 post-operative patients concluded that massage helped to reduce pain after an operation.

CHILDREN & MASSAGE

Touch and massage are increasingly being encouraged on children's wards. This not only benefits the children, it is also immensely therapeutic for the parents because it gives them something positive and truly useful to do, instead of sitting anxiously by their child's bed.

Research shows that touch is more effective than other types of comfort. In 1979, researchers at the University of Iowa looked at ways of alleviating stress and stopping crying in children. They compared the effects of stroking, patting, and holding, with verbally comforting sounds such as humming or soft talking. After five minutes, only 12 percent of the group listening to sounds had stopped crying compared with 88 percent of the children who had received comforting touch.

If your child is finding it difficult to settle in hospital, try smooth, rhythmic strokes along his back while he is lying on his front. Gently knead the shoulders and then use cat strokes (*see pages 30–31*) down his back. Your child need not undress – you can massage through light clothes.

MASSAGING THE VERY ILL

When you massage someone who is very ill, as the eminent 19th-century French surgeon Lucas Championniere said, "Your hands should be little more than a caress." But even when the patient is extremely thin and fragile, and the massage is simply very gentle stroking, the effects can still be extraordinary. It is wonderful to see someone's breathing get deeper, to see the tension leave their face, and to feel their muscles beginning to relax.

Often, friends and relatives do not know what to do when they are visiting someone who is very ill. Massage seems especially beneficial at this time, because you can communicate through touch when words are no longer easy or appropriate. A hand massage is suitable because it does not disturb the patient. Alternatively, you could try massaging the shoulders, face, or feet.

MASSAGE IN HOSPICES

Massage is increasingly being used in hospices as a way of alleviating suffering and improving quality of life. One of the reasons that it is so beneficial is that the person is allowed to lie there and enjoy the massage without feeling that they should respond in any way. They can let go and luxuriate in the relaxing sensation.

Many hospices are teaching friends and relatives how to perform a simple hand or foot massage. Staffs say it can be a great help: relationships are strengthened as relatives are able to do something positive rather than just stand by feeling helpless.

It is amazing to see that, even when you are extremely gentle, massage can have a profound effect. For example, one elderly lady who was dying, surrounded by her family, could no longer communicate verbally. A massage therapist massaged her hand, which was tightly clenched and, when she finished, she felt the old lady squeeze her hand in thanks. This reassured the family that their relative could still recognize touch and hear what they were saying. For the next few hours they held or massaged her hand and talked of happy memories. The old lady died later that night. The family said that they had felt much closer to her as a result of touching; it made the situation easier to bear and they felt that they had helped her to die peacefully.

HELPFUL TREATMENTS

✦ *Hand massage* (see pages 60–61).
✦ *Self-massage* (see pages 48–61).
If you are stiff, try stroking, kneading, and pressing (see pages 20–39).
✦ *Shiatsu* (see pages 94–97). To reduce pain, headaches, and nausea, press the points on the hands and wrists.

❛ *Touch is a language of its own with a very large vocabulary. Through touch we can communicate what cannot be spoken, for it is the true voice of feeling.* ❜

ASHLEY MONTAGUE, TOUCHING, 1971

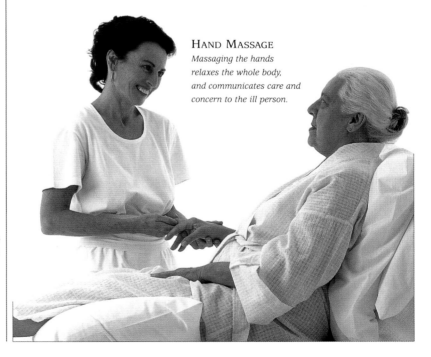

HAND MASSAGE
Massaging the hands relaxes the whole body, and communicates care and concern to the ill person.

THE ANATOMY

A KNOWLEDGE OF THE ANATOMY underpins the effectiveness of therapeutic massage. I believe that knowing how muscles are structured, and why they become sore, helps enormously when giving a massage. We can, for instance, tailor our strokes to mimic the way that blood is pumped into the muscles, thereby stimulating circulation and relieving stiffness.

THE MUSCLES

The muscles that are attached to the skeleton are "voluntary" muscles, meaning that we can control their movements. They are formed of hundreds, sometimes thousands, of muscle fibers that also contain blood vessels and nerves. The fibers are "wrapped" into bundles with connective tissue to form a muscle, which is further strengthened with an outer covering called a muscle sheath. Tendons attach muscles to bones, and are formed from the ends of the connective tissue and the muscle sheath.

PAIRS OF MUSCLES

We massage the body evenly for a good reason: muscles work in pairs and it is important that partner muscle groups receive equal attention. When we massage the upper arm, for example, we work on both the biceps and the triceps, which are situated on the front and the back of the arm respectively. These muscles work together to move the arm; to bend the elbow, for instance, the biceps contracts and the triceps relaxes and lengthens. To straighten the elbow, the process is reversed.

MUSCLE SORENESS

There are a number of reasons why muscles may become sore. Firstly, during exercise, in a process known as metabolism, muscles burn up a mixture of glucose and oxygen to release energy. The waste products (metabolites) that result, which include carbon dioxide, water, and lactic acid, are mostly

removed by the circulation, but they may build up in the tissues, causing transient pain.

Secondly, when muscles are inactive for a prolonged period of time, the connective tissue surrounding the muscle

fibers can shorten and become "stuck" to adjacent connective tissue. If a muscle is then exercised, microscopic tears may appear in the covering of the muscle, leading to inflammation and pain.

Finally, soreness can result if a muscle is habitually tense. When muscles are relaxed, blood can flow freely, but when they contract, the blood vessels within the muscles are squeezed. In time, the supply of blood to a permanently tight muscle will become impaired, and substances such as plasma, and calcium and other minerals may leak into it.

THE SKELETAL MUSCLES

The body has over 600 skeletal muscles. Each muscle is attached to two bones and, when it contracts, one bone moves while the other remains stable. The illustrations show the most common muscles that you will come across in massage.

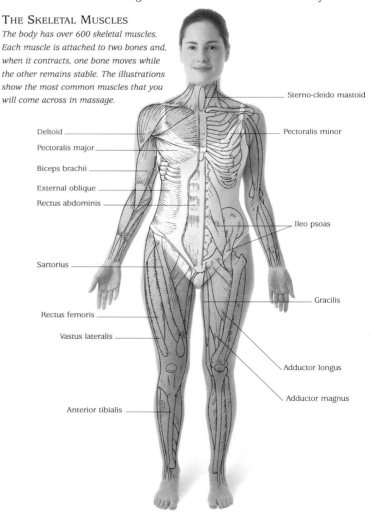

- Sterno-cleido mastoid
- Deltoid
- Pectoralis major
- Biceps brachii
- External oblique
- Rectus abdominis
- Pectoralis minor
- Ileo psoas
- Sartorius
- Gracilis
- Rectus femoris
- Vastus lateralis
- Adductor longus
- Adductor magnus
- Anterior tibialis

As a result, the muscle fibers can stick together and the connective tissue that wraps the muscle fibers may thicken, causing bunching of muscle fibers. The effect of these changes is to limit the affected muscle's range of movement.

EASING SORENESS

Mobilization of the muscles through gentle exercise helps to relieve soreness. Massage can also ease soreness because it relaxes taut muscle fibers and increases the local circulation, which helps to remove metabolites and other chemicals that cause pain and stiffness.

When you massage someone with habitually tense muscles, they may initially experience soreness and pain.

This is because, as well as helping to separate the fibers, deep pressure to bunched muscles may also cause microscopic tears to the connective tissue, resulting in inflammation and pain. In time, however, massage will help the muscle fibers to lengthen, separate out, and regain their movement.

THE NERVOUS SYSTEM

Massage has a powerful effect on the nervous system which, like a computer system controlling a complex machine, is responsible for second-to-second control of all aspects of the body. Depending on the strokes you use, you can stimulate or relax the body in moments.

The brain and spinal cord together form the central nervous system (CNS). The brain interprets information while the spinal cord acts as an information highway. Pairs of sensory and motor nerves connect the CNS to the rest of the body in the peripheral nervous system.

The sensory organs, such as the eyes, ears, and skin, relay information through the sensory nerves to the spinal cord and then to the brain, where it is interpreted. In response, the brain sends orders for action via the motor nerves to the appropriate part of the body.

Massaging the skin sends messages via the nervous system to the brain. Soothing strokes, for example, can act as a distraction and can induce a feeling of well-being and relaxation.

AUTONOMIC NERVOUS SYSTEM

What is known as the autonomic nervous system (ANS) controls internal functions such as blood pressure, respiration, heart rate, and digestion.

The ANS is composed of two parts: the sympathetic and the parasympathetic. They both control the same organs, but they have opposite effects. The sympathetic system stimulates body activity and becomes dominant during stress, anger, or exercise. If a car suddenly pulls out in front of you on the highway, you may feel your heart beating with extra force. This is a direct result of the sympathetic system stimulating the release of adrenaline to make your heart beat faster.

The parasympathetic system has the opposite effect. It allows the body to rest, so that digestion and other functions can take place. Relaxing during massage allows the body to rest, conserves energy, and helps the parasympathetic system.

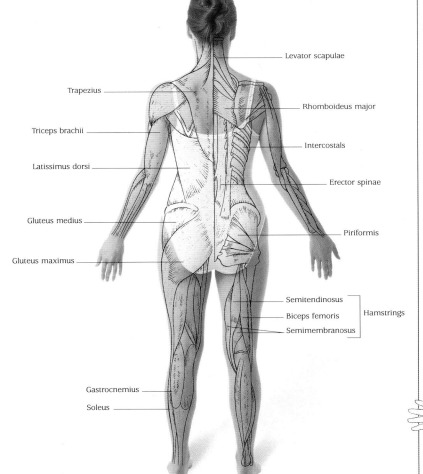

Levator scapulae

Trapezius

Triceps brachii

Latissimus dorsi

Gluteus medius

Gluteus maximus

Gastrocnemius

Soleus

Rhomboideus major

Intercostals

Erector spinae

Piriformis

Semitendinosus

Biceps femoris } Hamstrings

Semimembranosus

SENSORY NERVES
Shown here is the relative distribution of sensory nerves in the skin. The face, hands, and feet have far more nerve endings than the trunk.

THE CIRCULATION

One of the chief benefits of massage is its stimulating effect on the circulatory system, helping to improve the transport of oxygen and nutrients to individual cells, and assisting in the return of blood to the heart.

THE BLOOD

Essential for life, blood is composed of 45 percent cells and 55 percent plasma. Red blood cells carry oxygen and carbon dioxide, while white blood cells protect us from infection by making antibodies and by immobilizing and killing bacteria and viruses. Other cells, called platelets, help the blood to clot and are responsible for "plugging" minute holes in damaged blood vessel linings.

As the blood flows through the liver, it is enriched with glucose, amino acids, and other nutrients that the body needs for energy, growth, maintenance, and repair. The endocrine glands secrete hormones into the blood for transport to their target organs. The blood carries all these vital substances to the cells of the body.

THE HEART & BLOOD VESSELS

The heart is a muscular pump that is divided into left and right sides, each of which has two chambers: an atrium at the top and a ventricle at the bottom. Blood is pumped, first from the right ventricle to the lungs to be oxygenated, and then from the left ventricle to circulate around the body.

A complex web of blood vessels supplies blood to the tissues. The arteries, which carry blood away from the heart, have muscular, elastic walls that expand and spring back into shape following each heart beat to help them propel blood along at high pressure. Smaller vessels, arterioles, branch off from the arteries. They can dilate to take a greater volume of blood or constrict to take much less, and in this way they control blood flow and help to regulate blood pressure. From the arterioles, microscopic blood vessels called capillaries take blood to the cells.

They are semi-permeable, allowing water, oxygen, nutrients, hormones, and other substances to pass to the cells.

Blood is carried back to the heart in the veins, which have valves to prevent blood flowing backwards. Blood flows more slowly in the veins than in the arteries, and is assisted in its return to the heart by the action of the muscles.

IMPROVING THE CIRCULATION

Massage not only improves the flow of blood to the tissues: the squeezing, pumping actions of many massage strokes mimic the action of the muscles, helping to return blood to the heart. By massaging limbs in the direction of the heart, you can further assist this process.

THE LYMPHATIC SYSTEM

The lymphatic system has a dual role: it drains excess tissue fluid (lymph) back into the bloodstream (*see page 74*) and the lymph glands (the spleen, thymus gland, tonsils, and adenoids) produce lymphocytes which help to fight infection.

Lymph flows from the tissues into the initial lymph vessels, and then into larger lymph vessels, which have valves to maintain a one-way flow. Eventually the lymph drains into the subclavian veins of the neck, where it joins the blood circulation. Gentle massage, such as MLD (*see pages 74–77*), helps to stimulate lymphatic flow .

THE CIRCULATORY SYSTEM

In approximately one minute, blood completes a full circuit from the heart through the arteries (red) to the tissues, and back via the veins (blue) to the heart.

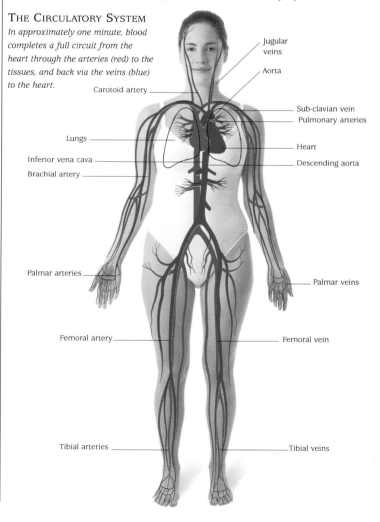

Jugular veins

Aorta

Carotoid artery

Sub-clavian vein

Pulmonary arteries

Lungs

Heart

Inferior vena cava

Descending aorta

Brachial artery

Palmar arteries

Palmar veins

Femoral artery

Femoral vein

Tibial arteries

Tibial veins

THE SKIN

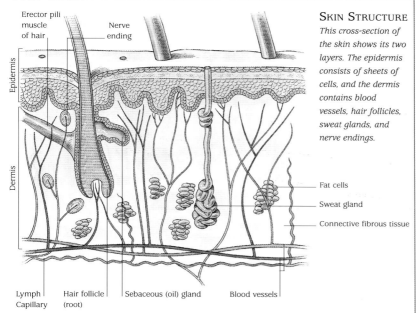

Erector pili muscle of hair

Nerve ending

Epidermis

Dermis

Lymph Capillary

Hair follicle (root)

Sebaceous (oil) gland

Blood vessels

Fat cells

Sweat gland

Connective fibrous tissue

SKIN STRUCTURE
This cross-section of the skin shows its two layers. The epidermis consists of sheets of cells, and the dermis contains blood vessels, hair follicles, sweat glands, and nerve endings.

The skin is the organ of touch, making it probably the most important organ of the body as far as massage is concerned. It is also the largest body organ, with an area of 5 to 6½ square feet and a weight of about 10 pounds. It is vital to life, keeping the body hydrated, protecting it from bacteria, and regulating its temperature.

The skin has two layers. The outer layer, the epidermis, is waterproof and can destroy bacteria. It contains melanin, which increases when stimulated by sunlight, and is one of three pigments responsible for differences in skin coloring. (Carotene and hemoglobin are the other two.) Vitamin D, necessary for calcium metabolism, is also made in the epidermis by the action of ultraviolet light on the skin.

The underlying layer, the dermis, contains nerve endings that sense touch, pressure, pain, and temperature. It is estimated that a square inch of skin contains 575 sensory receptors, making the skin extremely important for relaying information about our immediate environment to the brain. So sensitive are the sensory receptors,

that by adapting our massage techniques, it is possible to induce a wide range of feelings, from exhilaration to blissful relaxation.

The dermis also contains blood and lymph vessels, sebaceous glands that secrete sebum, an oily fluid that softens the hair and skin and destroys bacteria, and sweat glands, which help to control body temperature.

PAIN & MASSAGE

Pain is a protective mechanism that is essential for our survival. It makes us pull our hands away from a hot object to avoid injury, for example.

The sensation of pain is transmitted from pain receptors up the spinal cord to the thalamus in the brain. It is then transmitted to the sensory cortex, which interprets where the pain is located.

There are two types of pain: acute pain, which is the sharp, localized pain you experience when you prick your finger, and chronic pain, which varies from being a dull ache to severe, persistent pain.

Acute pain is unpleasant but short-lived. It is usually more difficult to cope with chronic pain because the cause can be difficult to pinpoint. It can last for years, and it can profoundly affect our everyday lives. When this type of pain persists, people often feel helpless and suffer from depression, anxiety, insomnia, and fatigue.

There are many factors that affect perception and tolerance of pain. Our expectation of pain, anxiety level, previous experiences, and ability to cope, as well as our ethnic origin, age, and general physical condition may all have a bearing on how we cope with pain.

THE GATE THEORY

The Gate Theory of Pain, first outlined by Melzack and Wall in 1965, proposed that there is a mechanism, or "gate," that limits the number of impulses that are transmitted up the spinal cord to the brain at any one time. According to the theory, nerves carrying the sensation of light, touch and pressure, transmit their impulses faster than the nerves that carry information from pain receptors. The theory helps to explain how, in this way, massage can ease pain.

If you rub your elbow after you have hurt it, the rubbing action usually helps to relieve the pain. This is because the sensation of rubbing the skin reaches the gate in the spinal cord first. The gate will then be closed to the pain impulse because another impulse (rubbing the skin) is already being transmitted to the brain. In this way, massage, as an alternative stimulus, should help to close the gate to pain impulses.

As well as acting as a distraction, massage induces relaxation, diminishes arousal, and gives a feeling of well-being. It also temporarily increases the local circulation, removing substances released by injured tissues (histamine, prostaglandins, and lactic acid) that can sensitize the pain receptors. All of these actions help to reduce perception of pain.

RESEARCH & BIBLIOGRAPHY

RESEARCH

PREGNANCY, BABIES & CHILDREN

✦ Acolet et al., "Changes in plasma, cortisol and catecholamine concentrations in response to massage in pre-term infants," *Archives of Disease in Childhood*, 68 (1993), p. 29–31.

✦ T. Field et al., "Massage reduces anxiety in child and adolescent psychiatric patients," *Journal of American Academy of Child and Adolescent Psychiatry*, 31 (1992), p. 125–31.

✦ T. Field et al., "Tactile kinesthetic stimulation effects on pre-term neonates", *Pediatrics*, 77, 5 (1986), p. 654–658.

✦ Ongoing research on massage, babies, and children, Touch Research International, University of Miami School of Medicine, Miami, Florida.

✦ K. Wheldall, K. Bevan & K. Shortall, "A Touch of Reinforcement: the effects of contingent teacher touch on the classroom behavior of young children," *Educational Review*, 38, 3 (1986).

MASSAGE FOR SPORTS

✦ B. Balke, Anthony & Wyatt, "The effects of massage treatment on exercise fatigue", *Clinical Sports Medicine*, 1 (1989), p. 189–196.

✦ Jordan & Jessup, Study on muscle strength, University of North Carolina, *Massage Therapy Journal*, (Winter 1990), *Understanding Sports Massage*, ed. Benjamin & Lamp, 1996.

✦ A. N. Rinder & C. J. Sutherland, "An investigation of the effects of massage on quadriceps performance after exercise fatigue," *Complementary Therapies in Nursing and Midwifery*, 1 (1995), p. 99–102.

✦ Smith et al., "The effects of athletic massage on delayed muscle soreness, creatine, kinase and neurophil count," *Journal of Orthopedic and Sports Physical Therapy*, 19, 2 (1994), p. 93–99.

STRESS & INSOMNIA

✦ T. Field et al., "Massage reduces anxiety in child and adolescent psychiatric patients," *Journal of the American Academy of Child and Adolescent Psychology*, 31, 1 (1992), p. 125–131.

✦ Jodo et al., "Effects of facial massage on spontaneous EEG," *Tohoku Psychologica Folia*, 47 (1988), p. 8–15.

✦ Levin, Stress induced in healthy volunteers, University of North Carolina, 1990.

✦ J. Longworth, "Psychological effects of slow stroke back massage in normotensive females," *Advanced Nursing Science*, 4, 4 (1982), p. 44–61.

✦ McKechie et al., "Anxiety states; a preliminary report on the value of connective tissue massage," *Journal of Psychosomatic Research*, 27 (1983), p. 125–129.

✦ Weinberg, Jackson & Kolodny, "The relationship of massage and exercise to mood enhancement," *Sports Psychologist*, 2 (1989), p. 202–211.

HEADACHES

✦ Göbel, Schmidt & Soyka, "Effect of peppermint and eucalyptus oil preparations on neurophysical and experimental algesimetic headache parameters," *Cephalalgia*, 14, 3 (1994), p. 228–234.

✦ H. Kurtland, "Treatment of headache pain with auto-acupressure," *Diseases of the Nervous System*, 37 (1976), p. 127–29.

✦ K. Puustjarvi et al., "The effects of massage in patients with chronic tension headaches," *Acupuncture and Electro-therapeutic Research International Journal*, 15 (1990), p. 159–162.

ABDOMINAL COMPLAINTS

✦ P. Caan & N. Read, Research on irritable bowel syndrome, University of Sheffield, *Mind Body Medicine*, Consumer Report Books, 1993.

✦ Oleson et al., "Randomized, controlled study of premenstrual symptoms treated with ear, hand, and foot reflexology," *Obstetrics & Gynecology*, 82 (1993), p. 906–911.

✦ R. Sandler, Research on effects of stress on the abdomen, University of North Carolina, *Mind Body Medicine*, Consumer Report Books, 1993.

✦ Resenede et al., "A pilot study on the effect of exercise and abdominal massage on bowel habit in continuing care patients," *Clinical Rehabilitation*, 7 (1993), p. 204–209.

✦ W. Ueda et al., "Effect of gentle massage on regression of sensory analgesia during epidural block," *Anesthesia and Analgesia*, 76, 4 (1992), p. 783–785.

✦ W. Whitehead, "Gut feelings; stress and the G. I. tract," John Hopkins University School of Medicine, *Mind Body Medicine*, Consumer Report Books, 1993.

BACK PAIN

✦ D. Turk, "Chronic pain – new ways to cope," *Mind Body Medicine*, Consumer Report Books, 1993.

✦ T. Pincus, Study on arthritis and rheumatic diseases, Vanderbilt University School of Medicine, 1993

MASSAGE & THE ELDERLY

✦ J. Fraser & R. Kerr, "Psychological effects of back massage on institutionalized patients," *Journal of Advanced Nursing*, 18 (1993), p. 238–245.

✦ Langland & Panicucci, "Effect of touch on communication with elderly, confused patients," *Journal of Gerontology Nursing*, 8, 3 (1982), p. 152–155.

✦ D. Norfolk, "Challenge of the third age," *International Journal of Alternative and Complementary Medicine*, (Jan. 1997).

✦ Project at the Central & Cecil Housing Trust, Age Concern, UK, 1996.

MASSAGE & ILLNESS

✦ Corner, Crawley & Hilderbrand, "Evaluation of massage on cancer patients," *International Journal of Pallative Nursing*, (1995).

✦ Field et al., Research on the effects of sexual abuse being lessened by massage therapy, *Journal of Bodywork and Movement*, 1, 1, 2 (1997), p. 65–69.

✦ Interview with Dr. Candace Pert, *Massage Therapy Journal*, 33, 4, (Fall 1994), p. 64–72.

✦ C. Stevensen, "The psychological effects of aromatherapy massage following cardiac surgery," *Complementary Therapies in Medicine*, 2 (1994), p. 27–35.

✦ "The effects of massage on anxiety and depression levels and on immune function," Touch Research International, University of Miami School of Medicine, Miami, Florida, 1995.

MASSAGE IN HOSPITAL

✦ Farrow, "Massage therapy and nursing care," *Journal Nursing Standard*, 4, 17 (1990), p. 47–50.

✦ A. Ferrell Torry & O. Glick, "The use of therapeutic massage as a nursing intervention to modify anxiety and the perception of cancer pain," *Cancer Nursing*, 16 (1993), p. 93–101.

✦ Hillardd, "Massage for the seriously mentally ill," *Journal of Psychosocial Nursing and Mental Health Services*, 33, 7 (1995), p. 29–30.

✦ Lynch et al., "The effects of human contact on the heart activity," *American Heart Journal*, 88, 2, p. 160–168; *Journal of Nervous and Mental Disease*, 158, 2, p. 88–99.

✦ Marin et al., "Post-operative pain after thoracotomy," *Revue des Maladies Respiratoires*, 8 (1991), p. 213–8.

✦ McCaffery & Wolff, "Pain relief using cutaneous modalities," *Hospice Journal*, 8 (1992), p. 121–153.

✦ Triplett & Arenson, "The use of verbal and tactile comfort to alleviate stress in young hospitalized children," *Research in Nursing and Health*, 2, 1, p. 17–23.

✦ Van der Riet, "Effects of therapeutic massage on pre-operative anxiety in a rural hospital," *Australian Journal of Rural Health*, 1 (1993), p. 11–16.

RESEARCH OBTAINABLE FROM:

✦ The Research Council for Complementary Medicine, 60 Great Ormond Street, London WC1N 3JF, England.

✦ Touch Research International, University of Miami School of Medicine, P. O. Box 016820, Miami, Florida, USA.

✦ The Aromatherapy Database, Essential Oil Research Consultants, 2 Ruelle du Terte Butêt, 54230 St. Germaine le Guillaume, France.

BIBLIOGRAPHY

✦ Asokananda, *The Art of Traditional Thai Massage*, Duang Kamol, 1996.

✦ Asokananda, *Thai Traditional Massage*, Duang Kamol, 1996.

✦ A. Auckett, *Baby Massage, the Magic of the Loving Touch*, Thorsons, 1982.

✦ M. Beck, *Milady's Theory and Practice of Therapeutic Massage*, Milady, 1994.

✦ P. Benjamin & S. Lamp, *Understanding Sports Massage*, Human Kinetics, 1996.

✦ H. Benson, *The Relaxation Response*, New York Times Books, 1984.

✦ H. Benson, *Timeless Healing*, Simon & Schuster, 1996.

✦ C. Beresford-Cooke, *Shiatsu Theory and Practice*, Churchill Livingstone, 1996.

✦ M. Cash, *Sport and Remedial Massage*, Ebury Press, 1996.

✦ *Chinese Massage*, Shangai College of Traditional Chinese Medicine, 1990.

✦ *Chinese Massage Therapy*, Anhui Medical School, trans. H. M. Lee & G. Whincup, Routledge & Kegan Paul, 1983.

✦ *Chinese Massage Therapy*, Shangong Science and Technology Press, 1990.

✦ S. Fritz, *The Fundamentals of Therapeutic Massage*, Mosby Lifeline, 1995.

✦ D. Goleman & J. Gurin, *Mind Body Medicine*, Consumer Report Books, 1993.

✦ G. Inkeles, *The New Massage*, Allen & Unwin, 1980.

✦ W. Johnson, *The Anatriptic Art*, Simpkin Marshall, 1866.

✦ Y. Jwing-Ming, *Chinese Qigong Massage*, YMAA Publication Centre, 1992.

✦ J. H. Kellogg, *The Art of Massage*, Modern Medicine Publishing Co., 1929.

✦ D. Kreiger, *Therapeutic Touch*, Prentice Hall Press, 1979.

✦ F. Leboyer, *Loving Hands*, Knopf, 1976.

✦ L. Liddlell, *The Book of Massage*, Ebury Press, 1984.

✦ C. Maxwell-Hudson, *Aromatherapy Massage Book*, DK Publishing, 1994.

✦ C. Maxwell-Hudson, *The Complete Book of Massage*, DK Publishing, 1988.

✦ C. Maxwell-Hudson, *Pocket Massage for Stress Relief*, DK Publishing, 1996.

✦ P. McNamara, *Massage for People with Cancer*, The Cancer Support Center, Wandsworth, 1995.

✦ J. Mennel, *Physical Treatment by Movement and Massage*, J. & A. Churchill, 1945.

✦ A. Monatagu, *Touching, the Human Significance of the Skin*, Harper & Row, 1978.

✦ T. Namikoshi, *Shiatsu*, Japan Publications, 1972.

✦ R. Ornstein & D. Sobel, *Healthy Pleasures*, Addison Wesley, 1989.

✦ K. W. Ostrom, *Massage and the Original Swedish Movements*, Octagon Press 1991.

✦ C. Pert, *Molecules of Emotion*, Simon & Schuster, 1997.

✦ B. Ravald, *The Art of Swedish Massage*, Bergh Publishing Group, 1982.

✦ V. Schneider, *Infant Massage*, Bantam Books, 1979.

✦ M. Sinclair, *Massage for Healthier Children*, Wingbow Press, 1992.

✦ T. Stretch-Dowse, *Lectures on Massage and Electricity*, John Wright & Co., 1906.

✦ F. Tappan, *Healing Massage Techniques*, Appleton & Lance, 1988.

✦ Vercammen, *Oriental Medicine*, Serindia Publishing, 1995.

✦ A. Vickers, *Massage and Aromatherapy*, Chapman & Hall, 1996.

✦ H. & G. Whittlinger, *Introduction to Dr. Vodder's Manual Lymph Drainage*, Haug Publishers, 1982.

✦ Wood & Becker, *Beard's Massage*, Saunders, 1981.

INDEX

ACKNOWLEDGMENTS

AUTHOR'S ACKNOWLEDGMENTS
I would like to thank everyone who has so kindly helped with this book, especially the following people: Amina Shah, Gill Whitworth and Pat Williams for all their help and encouragement; Kira Balaskas for her help on the Thai massage section; Philip Beach for his help on the Chinese section; Carola Beresford-Cooke for her help on the shiatsu section; Lorna Dixon for her help on the aromatherapy section; Tim Goullet for his help on the sports section; Jackie Pietroni for her help on the anatomy, physiology and medical sections; Anne Vadgama for her help on the Manual Lymph Drainage section; my clients, patients, students and teachers for all that they have taught me over the years; everyone at Dorling Kindersley, especially Nell Graville, Carole Perks, Monica Chakraverty, Toni Kay, Tracey Clarke, and

Krystyna Mayer; and finally, Sandra Lousada, both for all her enthusiasm, and her beautiful photographs.

PUBLISHER'S ACKNOWLEDGMENTS
DK Publishing would like to thank: Kira Balaskas, Phil Beach, Tim Goullet, and Anne Vadgama for their help with the Masterclasses. Thanks to Penny Warren for her help on Massage for Health, and to Brightside, Lightbox, Marianna Sonnenburg and Bridget Peirson.
Artwork John Woodcock and Lydia Umney.
Models Abdul Ahmed, Gustavo Aranha, Amanda Bibby (Close), Stuart Binns, Salima Hirani; Laura Jackson, Heli Kauppila, Kate Loustau (Close), Emy Manby, Inigo Manby, Susannah Marriott (and Olive), Amina Maxwell-Hudson, Jacqueline Phillips, Tim Pilcher, San San (MOT), Rachana Shah, Jo Smith, Laura Steinhart, Pollyanna Stokoe, Kaz Takabatake,

Mark Teversham, Kwong Tse.
Make-up Artists Amanda Clarke, Barbara Jones, and Jayne Robinson (Artistic Licence).
Picture Credits The publisher would like to thank the following for their kind permission to reproduce their photographs. Key: t = top; b = bottom; l = left; r = right; c = center. AKG London, 100tl; Axiom Photographic Agency, 74tl; Bridgeman Art Library, 82tl; Andy Crawford, Steve Gorton & Gary Ombler, 6tl, 10tl, 85cl, 112br, 118cr, 121cl & br, 128cr, 153tr; Mary Evans Picture Library, 96tl; Tim Ridley, 14; The Wellcome Institute Library, 70tl.

MASSAGE COURSES
For details send a stamped self-addressed envelope to The Clare Maxwell-Hudson School, PO Box 457, London, NW2 4BR. Website: www.cmhmassage.co.uk